HEAL THYSELF
For Health and Longevity

QUEEN AFUA

A&B BOOKS PUBLISHERS
Brooklyn, New York
11201

Library of Congress Catalog Card No: 91-72476
ISBN 1-881316-01-7 (Paper)
ISBN 1-881316-50-5 (Cloth)

Typesetting and editing by:
Sababu N. Plata of African World Infosystems

Assistant editors: Carol Daugherty, Shirley McRae, Gerianne
F. Scott and Naikyemi S. B. Odedefaa (Cheryl J. Sneed)
Hru Ankh Ra Semahj Se Ptah

Photographs by Anthony Mills.
Principal Models: Ayodele Martin Aubert, Nalanie Hope and
Najami Lezma.

The contents of this book are merely for the
purpose of education and information. This book is *not*
intended to serve as a substitute for medical supervision

A&B BOOKS PUBLISHERS
149 Lawrence Street
Brooklyn, New York 11201
(718) 596-3389

Second Printing 1992

HEAL THYSELF

For Health and Longevity

QUEEN AFUA

"...you have the power to create in your life what you want it to be. Purification is the key. Within this natural way of living and being, I choose not to cut, nor radiate, or drug my diseases away. Instead, I wash, pray, fast juice and bless my Dis-ease away."

Queen Afua

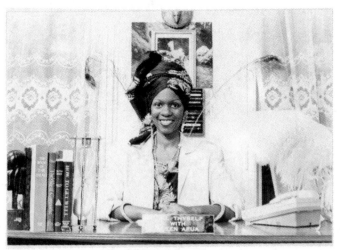

About the Author

Queen Afua is the founder and director of the Heal Thyself Center which was established in 1982. She, with the help of a dedicated staff, has guided over 10,000 people onto and through the path of purification with various natural systems of self-healing. Thousands have been guided through the 21-Day Urban Living Fasting Program she has created.

Queen Afua is also the founder and director of "Sacred Women," a nine hour intensive training on how to be a Full Woman and a Healed Woman for self, nation and world building. With Queen Esther she is co-founder of the original Sister to Sister Support Group, since 1988, which was also served by Lady Prema with her crystals and her prayer work.

Queen Afua is a certified colon therapist, certified polarity practitioner, holistic health consultant, Bach flower therapist, lay midwife, herbalist and fasting specialist. She has appeared on several television and radio talk shows.

The Heal Thyself Natural Healing Method is a loving vehicle that will give a greater number of people the opportunity to heal themselves. For total health, we must accept natural living and fasting as a way of life and as a way of acquiring healthy habits for longevity.

Contents

CONTENTS

CONTENTS

CONTENTS

Preface

The healer differs from the medical doctor in that the medical doctor is a learned and trained technician in methods for alleviating systems of illness that may or may not be part of his/her personal experience. The healer is someone who has through his/her personal experience learned to utilize life's obstacles for growth and development. When through understanding trial and error an obstacle, problem or illness is overcome and a new experience of benefit is born out of an old problem, true healing has taken place.

When such an individual extends his/her healing experience to others to help guide them through what they have experienced, a healer is created. The process is continual. As the healer helps to guide others he/she too is guided from within on the path of evolution.

In 1979, I had the pleasure to meet such an individual in the person of Queen Afua. A year later, I was to witness the opening of the Heal Thyself Natural Living and Education Center.

Since that time she has been my mentor and inspiration on the journey to health. Through the years I have been irrigated, steamed, bathed, "herbed," "fasted" and "clay packed" by the Queen.

Presently I can testify the most powerful healing agent of this extraordinary person is the Queen herself.

At the time of this writing, I had the pleasure of being worked on by Queen Afua. She was about to apply a healing agent to my body when right before application the congestion in my chest began to break up and disperse This was quite an extraordinary experience, I might add.

Prepare yourself, for this is no ordinary book. You have in your hand excerpts from a journey to "holiness." The light that channels through the author onto the following pages is a love offering to your health. Read and Be Well.

Dianna Pharr

About The Book

Bob Law announced on WWRL Radio Station, August 1990, that Queen Afua is writing a book. I had not begun to think about writing, but once I got over the shock of this community announcement I looked at this as a last spiritual command and message from the Creator to write down my sixteen years of acquired knowledge in Natural Healing and Fasting.

So I began to write and write and rewrite until August 1991, at which time the first edition of *Heal Thyself For Health and Longevity* was born out of me. It was not an easy birth but the baby is healthy and strong with the help of my editors.

In the words of Bob, "The future offers each of us significant challenges and opportunities. We can simply repeat our past experiences or we can explore new levels of awareness. We can chart a flight-plan for success."

This book is a manual for the future. It contains ideas that can help each of us reinvent our lives. I believe God wants us to constantly improve on the **gifts** that He has given us.

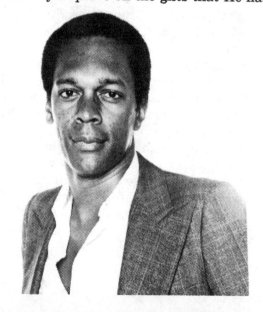

Dedication

I learned from my father that you are never too old to grow and heal. My father became a vegetarian at the age of 81 and together we put down his walking cane by following Natural Laws. At the age of 82, his arthritis left him and he jogged down the street. Sometimes at night, while I was reading to my father he would say, "I'm tired... I'm ready to leave this world now." With my innocence, enthusiasm and love, I would say, "Daddy, you are just a child in the eyes of God and you could live 100 years, like the folks you've read about in the Bible, if you live naturally."

Consequently, Daddy had become my best client and believer in healing. In his dying bed, my father sipped garlic juice I gave him. He touched my pregnant stomach, where my son Ali was living and said, "Helen, did you open the Healing Center yet?"

That was nine years ago. He didn't recollect my name very well, for by that time he was in both worlds and making his transition in a hurry, but he did remember my work and envisioned my destiny.

Every now and again when I don't know where to turn in my business affairs, my daddy comes from the spiritual world and gives me guidance. I want you to know Daddy, that I appreciate and enjoy those meetings.

So, to Ephraim Robinson, who believed in and raised me on long talks about Marcus Garvey, Martin Luther King and Malcolm X, who lectured on Black folks owning and operating their own businesses and working together for our salvation, I dedicate this book.

This book is also dedicated to my mother, Ida, who loves and supports my work, and my three children, Daoud, Sherease and Ali, who sacrifice with me in the effort to share the Almighty Creator's Purification Laws.

Acknowledgments

Most humbly, I give thanks to the Creator for giving me the desire, determination and support to heal myself and for the following people in my life: My mother, Ida, for being my best friend and confidante, and for helping me, along with my two brothers (James and Albert), to raise my children to be whole beings. Ah, my nine aunts, when I see them I get strength. They taught me the power of womanhood.

To my beloved friend, Bob Law, of "Night Talk" (WWRL RADIO), who consistently promotes healing throughout the land, and to his beautiful wife, Muntu, who lovingly propelled me to finish this book.

Elder Micah, the Godfather of Purification/Natural Healing, inspired me to create my formulas. Many thanks! Love to my sacred editors and literary midwives for diligently assisting in the birth of this work: Carol's faith, Gerianne's unrelenting push, Naikyemi's patience, and Shirley's love.

Love to Queen Esther, who stands to my right and demonstrates unconditional, lasting and noncompetitive love and for being the one who shared so much of my joy and some of my tears. I'm eternally grateful.

To Lady Prema, sacred songbird and spiritual "auntie," who stands to my left and always makes me mindful of the Creator's presence in my life.

To Cantor Cohen Nabiyim Deborah Yahbah for her divine prophecy about the expansion of my healing work.

To my spiritual reader and long-time friend, Dianna, whose readings have revealed to me my progress and life's lessons in a gentle way.

Much gratitude to my spiritual mother, Empress Akweke, for being the first to inspire me through her extraordinary lifestyle which lead me to be about the "Path of Purification." I give thanks to Empress Akweke for honoring me with the title "Queen." Love and Respect.

To my spiritual brother, Reggie Segars, who puts a song in my heart.

My most profound love and gratitude to my divine mate, Hru Ankh Ra Semahj Se Ptah, a present-day "King of Kings", for teaching me and so many others the ancient ways of our Khamitic ancestors, and for all those of the Temple of Ptah, who live and breathe our great and powerful legacy.

To Kalid, who shared the sounds of his golden flute with many fasters.

To the former staff of the Heal Thyself Center, the fasters, clients and students of the healing path who believed in themselves and the power of purification.

Healing and blessings to David Torain for "gifting" me with our three children who are my most precious gems.

To Richard Bartee, a gracious thank you for your continued support of the healing work.

Blessings to Benyamin for acting as co-Director of Heal Thyself from 1982 to early 1984.

To Rev. Philip Valentine who served as an instrument in protecting and ultimately saving my life and for acting as co-Director of Heal Thyself from late 1984 to 1988.

Immeasurable blessings to Imhotep Gary Byrd and Lloyd Strayhorn who supported me on my Natural Living Crusade throughout the years on the airwaves of Radio Station WLIB.

I salute Baba Ishangi, a masterful cultural teacher, world performer, healer and spiritualist who nursed me and thousands to the shores and through the waters to an Afrikan Beauty, Necessity and Reality.

Blessing to Hati Ast, a "Divine Mother,"whose love is as deep as life itself. To Mzuri, for allowing me to be silent, and for taking me (that winter's night) to the crossroads of my life when I didn't know quite where to turn. To you, a heart-felt embrace.

To Stevie Wonder, a shining light, who kindly allowed me to wrap him in herbs, for accepting my tonics and healing waters, and for capturing my heart with a song on my mama's piano... Love.

More love and healing to all the folks of the artistic world who continue to speak and dance and sing healing tones to our spirit, and for expressing deepest feelings in a way that inspires us all to flourish.

To all the Afrikan doctors, nurses and health professionals born in the Americas, the Caribbean, and across the globe, those who strive to heal our people, I offer my respect and adoration.

To all the holistic healers and naturopaths of the Four Directions who contain answers I don't have, I honor you. May the Creator continue to bless and protect you and your work.

To the indigenous Americans who maintain the sacred healing sweat lodges and who continue to perform the Sun Dance. Power and strength to your people.

Finally, to all those seeking to be healthy, happy and whole. May you have guidance and protection.

Introduction

History and Testimonial
MY PATH TO PURIFICATION

At the age of 17, I developed chronic asthma and severe hay fever. The road of health ignorance and darkness that I was traveling would have surely led to destruction had I not been rescued and led spiritually to the Path of Purification. I probably would have been living in an iron lung by now, had I survived at all.

There was no known cure for me according to the medical world. I was allergic to almost everything, grass, dust, fur, perfume, mold, several vegetables and fruits, and eggs, all of my life. In fact, the specialist that I was seeing told my mother that I was allergic to so many things that I really needed to live in a glass house. Even though I was getting my weekly injections and medication, as well as living on a special diet, I was becoming progressively worse.

How it all began is vivid in my mind. It was the evening of August 10th, 1970 at about 8:35 p.m. I sat with my family at the dinner table to partake of a "normal" meal of broiled steak, boiled potatoes with butter, muffins and collard greens. For dessert, I had a slice of cake and a glass of milk. I remember the meal being so heavy that after eating it I lost all of my energy and had to go to bed immediately. (I later had to outgrow the bad habit of "eating and sleeping" in order to heal myself.)

Ten minutes into my nap, I was awakened by my gasping for breath. My lung closed down; my face began to swell. I remember hearing myself say, "No air can get in or out." I was petrified; it was a labor to gain another breath. I thought, "I am going to die." I cried out, "Daddy, help me! I can't breathe!"

My father held my hand through the night during the bout of sickness, the first of many attacks to come. The word "attack" was so appropriate for I could feel an attack

1

on my mind, body and spirit. It was a total assault and there was nowhere to run.

I was an asthmatic! Every form of medication was given to me, but nothing helped. I deteriorated. I had to learn to live in a suffering state. This disease consumed my young life. Had not my mother told me I'd be alright and that people did not die anymore from asthma I don't know what would have happened to me then. Of course she was trying to comfort me, for I found out later that people do die from this respiratory disease. It was my belief in my mama's words that carried me and enabled me to clutch onto life. For when evening attacks came I remember I clung onto her words of hope for dear life. I felt that was all I had to hold onto. I would repeat in my mind my mothers's words that I was going to make it to dawn. "I am going to make it through the night 'cause you said I would, and I believe you mama. I have faith in you." For me, the closest person to God was mama and thus mama always told me the truth — and I believed her truth.

Many a night the asthmatic attack was so extreme that I would turn on the night light secretly so as not to disturb the rest of the household, and prop up several pillows against the sofa so I could quietly sleep sitting up all night, and for eight hours of pain and tightness in my chest I would wheeze a lot, sleep a little and pray, as I sat in fear of the next breath being my last. This inner turmoil would go on till the crack of dawn, for just as the sun was coming up so too my breath (life) would return — a quiet miracle. Once again, by the Creator's grace and my faith in my mama's words I survived another night.

My deepest disappointment was when I was told by my doctor that it would be impossible for me to take my scheduled college trip to Afrika. He predicted that I would become very sick in the grass and trees of my lost but not forgotten Motherland.

I did not yet understand that it had been my American meat-and-potatoes diet that had prevented me from being able to go home to Afrika. I had not made the connection between my diet and my health, so I continued to live in this ignorance and poor health for some time.

Three years went by. During these years, I developed arthritis in my shoulder as well as eczema all over my body. Later, I learned that these problems were a result of bad diet, inner rage, depression and not feeling able to express things I needed to express. When we heal we must be prepared to heal physically, mentally, emotionally and spiritually. We want complete healing.

One summer, a close friend invited me to a vegetarian retreat where I met the famous late great Afrikan American Master Herbalist for 50 years, Dr. John Moore, who later became my spiritual grandfather.

Three days before the retreat, I threw away my medication because I was feeling like a junkie who had to take legal drugs to stay alive. Deep in my soul I prayed that there was another way.

On my arrival at the retreat site, I saw grass and trees. I had no medication; I panicked. Thirty minutes later I began to wheeze; my eyes became red and bloodshot; my skin began to itch. I felt trapped. "What am I going to do now," I thought.

A quiet voice inside of me said, "Eat only lemons, grapefruits, and oranges and drink warm water." I did this for 28 hours, and all of a sudden, mucus was being expelled from everywhere, my eyes, nose and mouth. After about 24 hours of releasing in this way, I was able to breathe normally. My eyes became white, my skin stopped itching, and I was emotionally at peace.

For the remainder of the retreat I listened ecstatically to Dr. Moore and other lecturers speak on Natural Healing and Nature Cures. A whole new world opened for me. I realized that with faith, determination and a cleansed body temple, I could finally be healed.

Today, eighteen years later, I am disease-free. I continue to heal myself daily, and joyfully. My healing made me realize with the Creators grace and blessings that my people, and others who choose nature, no longer have to suffer and that freedom, spiritual, physical and emotional, is at hand.

These last 16 years I have been led on a crusade to teach and preach "Liberation Through Purification." I have learned to use every lesson as a blessing. My recovery from my illness gave me the determination to support thousands through their healing. My illness that turned to a healing has served as a catalyst for the "resurrection of a people."

l do not claim these writings to be the whole story on healing. The other part is within you, other healers and "would be" healers. However, the portion I'm led to share comes from my heart. Take this and use it wisely.

Glory be to the One Most High.

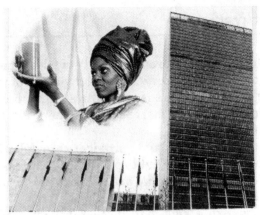

Chapter 1

A Cry For World Healing

Every nation shall read this book as a guide to natural healing — from the Continents to the Poles

This is a call for planetary healing and purification. A global resurrection is mandatory if we are to continue to thrive on earth.

This is a call to the United Nations, to the communities of the world. This is a call to our leaders — political, spiritual, educational, business and artistic — who have an even greater responsibility to purify, lest the people be led to mass destruction.

We have come into the age when our cleansing is most urgent, right here, right now. According to how we disrespect or respect nature and our body temples we will experience total devastation and destruction, or total enlightenment and resurrection. From the global to the personal, there is evidence that the necessity for the purification of the heart, mind and body temple is at an all-time high.

There is bloodshed due to wars. There are increased numbers of crimes in the streets. There are homicides and overcrowded jails. There are battered wives and abused children. There are the slow-death addictions and abuses of drugs and alcohol. There are out-and-out suicides. There is the soaring number of cancer victims and victims of the AIDS epidemic (plague). There is premature aging, heart attacks, hysterectomies and mastectomies. There are far too many "crib deaths."

With mental, spiritual and physical breakdowns everywhere, there is no choice but to purify. The rich, poor, young and old must cleanse if we are going to rise above the diseases of the body, mind and soul.

The Earth is expressing her discontent with how humankind has worked against natural laws. Ultimately, we have worked against ourselves. Our impure thoughts and acts of hate, rage, jealousy, depression and despair have led to the production of impure waters, acid rain, drought, devitalized soil and poisonous air. Equally, our bodies are filled with waste, worms and poisons.

Mother Earth warns us with her earthquakes, hurricanes and volcanic eruptions. Through fire and water, she is cleansing herself of all the filth, just as a woman cleans her womb of tumors by the fire of life-giving foods and water cleansings.

All religious and holy people and ancient spiritual masters of days gone by have shown us the truth and the way; that the foundation for liberation is to fast, to pray and to purify. The ancient masters did not eat of the flesh. They were vegetarians. They were clean.

We too must now walk in their footsteps. This way of living holds all the keys for peace on earth, for self-realization, success, health and resurrection for the healing of the planet and humankind.

We must cease our internal and external wars with ourselves and with one another. We must seek to live with a fervor and determination to expunge disease which runs rampant on this planet due to our unnatural lifestyles, greed and ears deafened to our own inner voices.

Early one morning, the Creator spoke through my inner voice: "Worry not, my children. Man does not control his destiny, I do. Refocus your eyes. Follow my ways, follow my laws and I will set you free!"

In response to my inner voice and in response to the Creator, I offer the following pledge:

I, Queen Afua, born Helen Odel Robinson, am reaching back into the beginning of time and drawing the strength, power and dignity of those ancient times and ancient folks. I affirm for my people and all people right here and now that our personal, spiritual and physical liberation is through purification. All I am able to reach I will share this Freedom call — "Liberation through Purification!"

My work and this book are attempts to right some of our wrongs, to give us formulas that help us go beyond mere survival in the coming age.

To my human family I say: Put the plate down, my sisters and brothers, my mothers and fathers. Let us fast and pray our way out of bondage and darkness into truth and light. Be victorious for our lives, our souls because our children's children lives and souls depend upon our purification. Glory be to the One Who Rules the Heavens and the Earth. It was true then as it is true now: *Physical, Mental and Spiritual Liberation Comes Through Purification.*

Let us liberate ourselves from disease and spiritual unrest. Peace can exist on earth, but it must with you. From you comes family healing, then community healing, national healing, and finally, global healing.

We must use the Creator's tools to heal ourselves. The tools are fasting, prayer, herbs, juices and live sun-ripened foods. We must maintain high and clean thoughts and allow divine, righteous love to flow through every cell so that we may build body temples of light.

Only the light beings will make it through; only the "shining" ones. These are a chosen few. Are you one of them? Wake up and rise into a Natural, Divine Way of Living so that you can *Heal Thyself*.

WHO AND HOW CAN I BENEFIT FROM THE HEAL THYSELF HOLISTIC HEALTH PLAN?

Who	Benefits
The Athlete	Develop more stamina and endurance. Control breathing and acquire stronger, cleaner lungs. Increase concentration. Become physically more flexible.
The Artist	Become more creative. Increase energy. Produce an effective stage presence. Increase your natural radiance and beauty. Singers range will be higher and deeper; the voice will be fuller.
The Business person	Reduce or eliminate stress. Develop brain power. Increase memory. Aid movement up the corporate ladder. Draw money and positive, successful contracts towards you.
Seekers of physical beauty	Experience weight loss. Rid your body of cellulite. Clear skin of acne, etc. Remove bags from under the eyes. Remove wrinkles and lines. Become poised and relaxed. Stimulate hair growth. Remove body odors. Acquire a pleasant speaking tone.
Lovers and mates	Experience more sexual fulfillment, and more intense orgasms.

Become more loving, gentle and in tune to yourself and with your mate.
Acquire spiritual awareness during lovemaking.
Have the ability to experience lovemaking as a sacred divine gift.

Your body will taste delicious. *Note:* Watch with whom you make love. Be sure that they cleanse for "we are what we eat."

The Family | Share in a healthy, progressive, strong and loving family unit.

Parents-to-be | Cleanse for three months to a year before you try to conceive. You will create a genius child, a love child, a disease-free baby. Many children are born today with cancer, retardation, arthritis, etc. Deep cleansing and rejuvenation before conception may prevent the occurrence of these illnesses.

Parents: Mothers and Fathers | Increase levels of patience.
Deepen love.
Increase energy levels.

Elders | Lessen aches and pains.
Decrease tendency toward senility.
Increase energy.
Experience a reversal of the aging process and increase physical power and strength.
Decrease the need for medications.

Know that life is not over, it's just beginning.

Spiritual life naturally seekers	Your prayer life will increase effortlessly. Temptations in the form of drugs or alcohol will be removed from you. Experience peacefulness and a greater capacity to have divine love. Have a closer relationship with the Creator. Your "third" eye (spiritual center) will open.

Chapter 2

Let The Healing Begin

As I stand on the island of Jamaica looking out on the Caribbean Ocean, I speak through my moving meditation. The curtain of the world opens and there are drums and shekeres being played in the background of the heavens. There is gospel music playing. "Hail to the Most High" is spoken.

I come out on the stage of life and say, "I've come to share with you a gift of healing, not simply because I'd like to but because I have to. Not because I want to, but because I need to.

You see, contained in this *Urn* (book) is gold dust, a magical gold that is within us. Whenever we are ready to heal, the gold dust becomes activated. The Creator has given us this inner gold by which to "Heal Ourselves." Once that inner gold becomes ignited and begins to shine, we become blissfully at peace and at one.

The healing begins to swell up within me and then I've got to share the feeling, because it's busting out of my toes and running through my fingers and pouring out of my eyes and exploding through my mind.

I've got to share this healing. My gold moves me to share this goodness. I've become so ecstatic about what the Creator has given us so magnificently through air, fire, water and earth that my joy has to be expressed through dancing about. But that isn't enough.

I have to sing about the healing and still that just isn't enough. Finally, I have to testify about my healing. So I jump for joy, get happy and shout. It has gotten so that I find myself thanking the Creator in every language. Hail to the Most High, Jah, Allah the Most Merciful, Jehovah, Olodumare, and Jesus because the healing is so full, so good, so massive it encompasses the world.

Oh, I've been delivered. I feel golden, just like the sun — always vibrating, radiating, glowing and sharing its light. That's why I've got to share my healing. I can't help myself. I love you too much not to share this good feeling.

In this magical *Urn* is all the gold that's inside of me. I'm going to sprinkle you down and God's going to lift you up. Ralph Carter! Lady Prema! Queen Esther! My Mama! My Daddy in the spirit world! And all my loves! LET THE HEALING BEGIN!

Many years have gone by, sixteen to be precise, and I've journeyed through the drama of our healing. I have talked to the elders about the healing, and taught the children about the healing. I've dried thousands of tears of women growing into their healing. I've massaged breast-feeding mothers, given counsel to the brothers, delivered beautiful babies. I loved my man through his healing. I've been through it all.

It seems the more I've gone through the more I'm feeling life, feeling free, feeling wonderful simply just to be. By way of my journey, I've purified myself so much until my third eye done opened. I'm getting a vision. I can see the world dancing, and healing, and shouting for joy. Fasters! Healers! Would-be Healers! There's a world healing going on. In all four corners of this earth there is a world healing going on, in the North, South, East, West. As I spread my hands throughout this universe in spirit, body, mind, and soul, I see in my inner vision a world healing going on. All war and destruction has ended. The mama within me and the father within me and within us have said, "There's a world healing going on." And so it is. Right now as we affirm together our healing, may the curtain stay open within your life and may the light of the Creator shine upon you and give you peace. For as sure as the sun sets and the moon rises, know that there's a world healing going on. It's going on within me, within you and within us. So let the healing begin!

Chapter 3

Prepare Yourself and Your Home

**Forgiveness and Thanksgiving are the
Keys to Spiritual Preparation for Healing**

As a spiritual preparation to embark upon the path of natural living and purification, we must be in a state of constant forgiveness so that we may be forgiven for the sins we have imposed upon ourselves and others. So let us affirm together: Today I forgive all the people, conditions and circumstances that ever hurt me in this life and past lives. For in my forgiving I begin the process of complete healing. The sickness within me is no more. Instead of holding onto anger, bitterness or sadness, I offer it all up to the Most High.

We must be in a state of thanksgiving for our many gifts and blessings. Let us give thanks and praise together: "I spread my arms to the north and south, and my heart to the east and west. I give full thanks and most gracious gratitude for my ancestors who laid the foundation for me to grow, to learn and to reach each beyond the stars. Thank you for showing me the way through the forest and trees. Thank you for being there in spirit. May I walk in your footsteps. May I one day become a wonderful and deserving ancestor."

"To our parents who were the avenues of our arrival to this earth: I love you, Mama and Baba (father). You gave me all you had to give and I give thanks. How much of my life can give you in return?"

To our mates, past and present: "You taught me my lessons of humanity, how to say yes and when to say no. You taught me the many levels of loving, the many levels of living and the many joys of forgiving."

To our children and the children of the world: "You have shown me how to love unconditionally, even when it was painful. Through my pain I had my greatest births, deepest understanding, and my most intense transformation. Glory, glory, glory.

"For the bird that flies past my window, the butterfly that has landed on my shoulder, the rain that falls and the sun that rises, I give thanks and gratitude to the Creator and to nature. Thank you for providing me with my healing continuously, freely, abundantly and lovingly." I give thanks in my hours of darkness and I give thanks in the light for each divine lesson given to me."

"I give thanks for each additional breath that I am given from the one who rules the Heavens and the Earth, my Great and Divine Mother Father." "I give thanks for my life, for giving and sharing life. I give thanks as I ecstatically look forward to all of life's challenges with joy and great expectation."

"Hail to the Most High for forgiveness and thanksgiving. Today, I bear witness to my complete healing. Forgiveness and thanksgiving flow through me. All of my sins are washed away."

Preparing the Home for Self-Healing

Your home is a reflection of who and what you are and the levels that you've reached in self-awareness. If your house is in order, your personal temple is usually at peace. On the other hand, if your home is out of order, there is usually some internal confusion or unrest within yourself.

Let's use this time to not only cleanse our inner temples but also to cleanse our outer temples. When you come in from the world and enter into your home, allow your home to be a sacred place, a place of refuge, a place where you can recharge, and gain balance and peace. Let it become a place to prepare you for your work in the world.

Clean out the old to make room for the new. Work within seven day cycles. Wash all floors. Use Florida water, ammonia, peppermint liquid soap. *Note*: One teaspoon cinnamon in the cleaning solution brings sweetness to your home.

- If you have an opportunity to paint your home or prayer room, then paint it.
- Clean out closets and drawers. They represent areas of your subconscious, your deepest, most hidden feelings which must be "cleaned out."
- Throw out all clothing and shoes which have only been gathering dust.
- Wash and press all clothing in an orderly fashion so that your mornings run smoothly and effortlessly. No last minute pressing clothes or looking for shoes. That's no way to go into work. If you leave your house scattered, you will find its reflection in the world.
- Open all windows in the house daily for a few moments during the winter months. During the summer months, keep the windows open for complete circulation of the air elements. Allow the air to constantly baptize you and lift you up high.

The Entrance To Your Home

Keep a vase full of fresh Lucky Leaves or a cactus plant near your doorway. You can also place three lemons over the doorway which you can change periodically. This is Dr. John Moore's spiritual formula to protect your home.

These natural elements spiritually aid in absorbing any adverse forces that are entering your home or will even better, repel them from coming into your sacred space. If you become very pure and holy then adverse forces will not enter or direct themselves toward your body temple or your sacred space. Negatives, as positives, are reflections. The body temple is the inner reflection and must be kept clean and your home is your outer reflection. It must be kept clean. Your thoughts must be purified for thought is the end result of your inner and outer life made manifest.

Helpful Hints about Colors

For best results when painting our home or even wearing colors on your body temple, remember these helpful hints about colors:

White	Purification
Violet/indigo	Spirituality and higher mind
Yellow	Peace and tranquility
Blue	Higher mind
Green	Healing
Soft Pink	Love
Orange	Stimulation
Red	Energy and Productivity

Your Home As A Healing Space

Living room

Avoid using the living room for constant video and television activity. Such activity creates dulled senses, slow thinking, and radiation poisoning, in most cases. Instead, use your living room as an opportunity for family communication, mediation, exercise or artistic expression.

Keep plenty of plants in the living room for greater oxygen supply. Additionally, have pillows so you can sit low. The low sitting causes flexibility in the body and humbleness in the spirit.

Your Kitchen as a Healing Laboratory

This area of the home is the foundation of higher health and healing to the entire household. The culinary chemist, whoever she or he may be, holds the physical, mental and spiritual blueprints of the family and future generations. The combination of nature's elements that we call food must be alive to give life, must be balanced to maintain balance within, must not be over-seasoned (which irritates) and above all, they must invigorate rather than stimulate. This room must be in total order. The state of mind is of paramount importance in this laboratory, for the emotional energy you entertain during the preparation of your food is the most important ingredient you contribute to the art. Your resulting formula can heal the household or destroy it.

Cleanse your refrigerator and discard all devitalized food. Their energies can pollute the nearby foods that have higher and more pure rates of motion, eg. fresh fruits and vegetables.

The following are further helpful hints to you, as chemist, on the make-up and maintenance of a powerful culinary laboratory.

Purification Kitchen Laboratory Tools

Juicer: Look for a good juicer to extract the juice from vegetables and fruits. Some juicers are not designed to extract the juice of oranges, grapefruits or lemons so you may have to purchase a citrus juicer or a special attachment for your juicer. A good juicer will separate the juice from the pulp. You can purchase a juicer at the local health food store or department store. If you can afford to do so, invest in a good one, such as Acme or Champion. The less expensive Oster vegetable and fruit juicer, which can be found in your local department store, is also suggested.

Blender: You can use a blender for mixing your nutrients in with your vegetable or fruit juices or for making fruit shakes and vegetable cocktails.

Measuring spoons and measuring cup: Carefully measure your nutrients, the waters for your tonics and the amount of juice you are required to take daily.

Sharp knife: Use to prepare fruits and vegetables for juicing. It is easier if the fruits and vegetables used are cut up into smaller pieces for juicing. It is also better for your juicer.

Cast iron, stainless steel, clay or glass pots; bamboo steamer: Avoid using aluminum utensils.

Strainer: A small mesh strainer is good for straining herbs from your health tonics and any excess pulp from your juices.

Garlic press: Purchase this only if you are going to use

fresh garlic cloves, instead of Kyolic, for your Kidney-Liver Flush.

Cutting board: Use this to prepare your fruits and vegetables for juicing.

Mugs and drinking cups: Have on hand 8 ounce, 12 ounce and 16 ounce drinking glasses for your juices and 12 ounce mugs for your Kidney-Liver Flush.

Large Mason jar: Use this to mix and steep your health tonics overnight.

Stainless steel or glass tea kettle: For boiling your water for your tonic and Kidney-Liver Flush.

Aloe plant: You may use this if you are a little out of tune, or get cut or burned while preparing the foods or herbs in your kitchen laboratory.

You may also want to put a sign over the doorway of your kitchen saying:

"_____'s Kitchen Laboratory."
(Write your name or family name above.)

Water Healing Supplies for your Hydrotherapy Room (Bathroom)

Whirlpool Bath	For circulation, healing and relaxing.
Water Pik	For localized water healing.
Enema bag (qt.)	For purging body temple.
Squatting stool	Squat on toilet to allow greater elimination.
Nose rinser: neti pot or kettle	For deeper, fuller breathing.
Loofah brush	To cleanse pores of skin.
Small candle	For quiet meditation (when in bath).

For atmosphere, add flowers, hanging plants, inspirational posters and sayings to beautify your hydrotherapy room. Make your bathroom beautiful and conducive to relaxation so that it can help you do the work of releasing poisons from your head to your toes. Peace should abound around the toilet, sink, shower, tub and all parts of your hydro-therapy room.

Toiletries

Oatmeal scrub	For soft skin.
Natural soaps	Afrikan Black soap, Clay soap, Peppermint soap, etc.
Bath oils	Eucalyptus and Peppermint oils.
Rosewater	For freshening up.
Almond oil	
Golden seal salve	
Vitamin E oil	For glowing skin.
Toothpaste	Use Queen Afua's Rejuvenating Clay for teeth and gums or Peppermint & Myrrh toothpaste.

Chapter 4

Dietary Timetable

When Should We Eat?

D*ietary Timetable* implies that there is a particular time during the day in which we can best handle food. Our body's energy level increases and strengthens as the sun gets stronger in the heavens, and decreases as the sun returns home (sets). Our body handles food according to the potency of the sun. If we desire ultimate health and longevity, weight loss and mental clarity, our dietary intake must reflect this in the amount and kinds of food eaten.

Sunrise

We should eat lightly because we are just coming out of a fast, that is, the 4-8 hours of non-eating that we spend sleeping. In the morning, we must not shock the body with heavy foods such as pancakes, meats, fried foods, rolls, etc. or even loud noises. We must gently rejoin body and spirit with a light diet, easy morning movement/exercise and with prayer and meditation. The lighter the sunrise "break-fast," the more in tune we can be spiritually. We will experience a greater energy level and be more mentally alert throughout the day. We should introduce foods into the body temple that are easier to digest like fruits and fresh juices. For those who are not satisfied with soya or nut milk, one piece of fruit and a cup of herb tea, such as chamomile (for the nerves), rosehips (vitamin C), or red zinger (relaxant and vitamin C) will suffice. If the mind is weak in the mornings, take 1 teaspoon of gota-kola herb tea with one cup of water, and steep for 30 minutes. For a "morning coffee" that's high in iron, add 3 table-spoons blackstrap molasses to a cup of warm water.

Sun Apex

By midday (lunch time), the sun is at its strongest point and so are we. Naturally, nutrition will be digested easier during this time. As a result, we should consume our heaviest meal during this time span. You can use the remainder of the day to exercise as a digestive aid for this midday meal. Such exercise could include walking, or running for the bus, walking stairs, and reaching and pulling with the arms. Exercise helps the body to quicken its pace in the acts of digestion, assimilation and finally elimination. Your body can have food such as proteins (soya meats, beans, peas, lentils, baked fish, nuts), complex carbohydrates (starches), steamed vegetables or raw salad. Study the food combination chart (provided later) for greatest digestion of your food. Note that all juices, teas, or water should be taken 30 minutes to 1 hour before or after your meal.

Sun Descent

By late day (dinner time), we are to eat light once again; for like the sun, we are to return home and allow the body to become quiet and light again. If we eat after the sun goes down, particularly heavy foods, we will suffer from indigestion, gas, nightmares, bad moods, weight problems and constipation. Food taken beyond the hour of sunset will ferment and poison the system even when the body is in a resting state.

In the Fall/Winter, your last meal should be taken between 4-5 p.m., but no later the 6 p.m., even if you have a late work night. In the Spring/Summer, the last meal should be taken between 7-8 p.m. If you must eat after preferable digestion hours then eat only fruits, fresh vegetables, salads, or drink fresh fruit or vegetable juices.

Within seven days of living according to the Dietary Timetable you will see a decrease in weight of 4-8 pounds and an increase in morning energy and power. Others will begin to notice that you have a beautiful morning disposition.

To move with the rhythm of the seasons, take note of the following:

Fall/Winter: We eat heavier foods to build heat in our bodies. We also hibernate (sit in) more. There is greater possibility for mental depression, aches and pains, shortness of breath, colds and fevers. During this season there is greater need for meditation, quiet movements and planning for the future (Spring-coming out).

Spring/Summer: We are ready to venture out into the world. We are more active. To keep up with the season, we eat lighter and naturally do more fasting. Act upon winter meditations. It is planting time!

To do any differently will cause our bodies to rebel by getting sick. Overeating, especially in the summer, causes tiredness, skin eruptions, high blood pressure, edema, etc.

Chapter 5

FASTING

What is Fasting?

There are various types of fasts, such as the water fast, fruit juice fast, wheatgrass fast, etc. The religious (spiritual) fast is the original fast. During a religious fast only water is taken into the body. In a "dry" religious fast, the food and drink is totally that of "the spirit."

In nature, when an animal is sick, it will fast until it is well, or it will eat only green grasses of the fields. When we humans are in harmony with ourselves, we also know to fast if we become unbalanced and need healing, or if we desire greater spiritual direction.

Sometimes when we become ill we eat crackers and chicken soup. Unfortunately, this is not a healing thing to do. At this time we should use a nutritional fasting method to heal and cleanse the body of poisons that have accumulated from eating meats, starches, sugar, cooked oils, and junk food. Sickness is the body's way of rebelling against disrespect and pollution.

There has also been disrespect for our environment. As a result the air we need to breathe and our waters are polluted. The earth that grows our food has been devitalized. Due to our disrespect of nature, the very elements we need for healing are in crisis condition, especially in the urban areas. We can no longer only drink water for survival as did the ancients. Even if we went to more rural areas in order to fast, we would experience violent detoxification crises due to our years of inner body pollution and dietary ignorance.

I have developed a nutritional fasting method that will cleanse the body temple with little or no stress to the body. I recommend freshly pressed fruit juices and purified or distilled water to purify, rejuvenate and strengthen the body. I also recommend specific vegetable juices as well as herbs (spirulina and wheatgrass), enemas, herbal laxatives and colonics. Healing baths and exercise are also major components of this fasting method. The body is fed all the necessary vitamins and nutrients. As a result, the oft-times uncomfortable cleansing reactions are lessened and you are able to maintain sufficient balance while both cleansing and leading your every-day life (family and home care, away from home occupations, study and school, etc.) You will experience emotional balance (unlike when on a strict water fast when you might experience mood swings or nightmares). The chlorophyll and vegetable juices aid in emotional harmony and physical strength. The fruit juices detoxify your various organs gently and lovingly.

Fasting... Who? Why?

Renew yourselves and fast, for I tell you truly, that Satan and his plagues may only be cast out by fasting and by prayer. Go by yourself and fast alone and show your fasting to no man. The living God shall see it and great shall be your reward. Fast 'til Beelzebub and all his evil depart from you and all the angels of our Earthly Mother come and serve you. For I tell you truly, accept fasting, or you shall never be freed from the power of Satan and from all diseases that come from Satan. Fast and pray fervently, seeking the power of the Living God for your healing.[1]

* * *

By fasting you will call back the Lord of your body and the angels. ... Each day that you continue to fast and pray, God's angels blot out each year of your evil deed from the books of your body and your spirit and when the last page is also blotted out and cleansed from all your sins, you stand before the face of the Creator pure and whole.[2]

After fasting, the body has purged the blood of toxins,

---

[1] Szekely, Edmond Bordeaux, ed. and trans. *The Essene Gospel of Peace* Book 1. International Biogenic Society, 1981.

[2] Ibid, pg. 29

clogging waste and decaying and diseased cells, then healthy cells are built of better material to replace those cast out of the body during the fast. That is regeneration. That is the Secret of the Ancient Masters. Know the law and observe it. That is the way to keep your body vigorous.

In the days of Adam and Noah, man ate only the juice of Fruits of nature and drank the water of coconuts. They ate less in a day, perhaps, than modern man eats in one meal. The duration of their youth extended over several centuries (Gen. 5:32), and they lived almost a thousand years.

The ancient masters recognized fasting as the great remedial measure and resorted to it in instances of illness. Fasting twice in the week was a common custom in the days of Jesus. The disciples of John fasted often. David fasted 40 days. Jesus fasted 40 days. Gandhi fasted to get the British out of India. These wise men knew how to promote health and prolong life and free themselves from bondage of any and all kinds.

Each day that you continue to fast and pray, God's angels blot out 1 year of your evil deeds from the book of your body and cleansed from all your sins, you stand before the face of God. (*Essene Gospel of Peace*, Vol. 1, p. 29) You must fast one day for each year that you've lived to totally purify yourself. Example: If you are 32 years old, then you should fast 32 days. If you are 26, then fast for 26 days and so on. Once you enter the kingdom of God through fasting, you receive prosperity, divine love, health, happiness and peace.

Purification for Spiritual and Physical Liberation

The one thing that all the religions have in common is "fasting and praying." This fasting and praying is to bring about liberation on every front. We, as a people, are governed by divine law. The highest law is fasting and prayer. If this is done diligently by the planetary members, the planet could function on a higher frequency and bring an end to pain and suffering.

Peace and harmony can occur on Earth but in order for this to occur we all must in our various religions and walks of life strengthen, double and quadruple our efforts at fasting. Fasting must come as a way of life. We should proceed with physical and spiritual haste due to the alarming conditions of the planet at this time.

Moslem fast: During Ramadan, a fast for 40 days in which they don't drink or eat until the sun sets.

Christian fast: On every Friday during Lent and on Good Friday, they don't eat or drink. Master fasters include Moses, Elijah, and Jesus (or Yeshua) who fasted for 40 days and 40 nights. Daniel fasted for 21 days and was a strict vegetarian. Blessings to Elder Micah, my godfather, for this information.

Jews/Israelites: They fast on a "Day of Atonement" once a year for repentance. The ancient Israelites ate only manna (a sea vegetable like spirulina/an algae from the ocean) for 40 years. They were not allowed to eat any meat.

Hare Krishna: The fast of Kadasi is done twice a month. For 24 hours one goes without water or sleep. One remains in a state of constant prayer and chanting. This is for the purpose of greater spiritual awareness and to be given more time to glorify God and to transcend the bodily demands. There are three other levels to their fast that are less intense. Blessing to HLA DINI SHAKTI, a devotee of Hare Krishna.

Indigenous American: This fast is done during general ceremonies, vision quest and the sun dance for the purpose of purification and healing. The fasting process varies from nation to nation. Blessings to Oscar Moreno, an indigenous American sweat lodge leader, for this information.

Yoruba Religious Fast

The New Year is a time for fasting. Fasting varies according to the faster's position in the community and what he/she are trying to achieve. Priests have the responsibility to foresee what must happen for the new period, so they go through a period of purification to be able to receive the holy messages. When they have achieved this period of "sacrifice" they have become lighter and one with the divine spirit. Most initiations have a period of fasting. The older you are, the longer you fast. Fasting is not only looked at as a cleansing but as a discipline, particularly for spiritualists who have to work long hours communing with the spirits. In various practices, it is a way to show the Divine in one's self, to remove one's self from the worldly pursuits.

Normally, during this kind of fasting a person withdraws and does a total fast, which means no social activity, no sexual intercourse. The person does take liquids and may only come out to take part in rituals. Everyone participating in the rituals looks towards those who have been in seclusion for the divine wisdom that comes as a result of their sacrifices. During the withdrawal period, the person is not just fasting, but praying and performing rituals. Often there are periods of chanting and singing. The person stays within an incubation state during which he/she hopes to receive the divine message.

Sometimes an *adept* will be allowed to come into the sacred area to record what the person might say in this trance-like state. Once the person awakes, the adept will inform him/her of everything that happened. The adept must be very wise because it is not only words for which they are listening. The prostrate body itself may get up and dance in a trance state and languages may come from the mouth that the adept has not heard.

The adept is also in a state of fasting, but has himself or herself on a more elementary level and has not secluded himself or herself as the other person has done. The reason for this is because the adept does not want to be charged up by the spiritual world and rendered unable to record the information from the one who is in the trance-like state.

Baba Ishangi
Yoruba Priest

Make fasting a way of life regardless of your own particular spiritual and/or cultural affiliation. Help to actualize miracles on earth.

When and Why to Fast

During your birthday month: In this month you will be receiving many messages on how to live out the coming year. Keep in mind that you are the ultimate spiritual reader of your own life. No one will know you better than you yourself and Almighty God the Creator. Fast and pray for all doors to open physically and spiritually.

Fast on your holy day: Fast 24 hours every week on your "holy day" or "Accra Day," which is the day of the week on which you were born.

Fast every seasonal change: To welcome in each season, fast 3, 7, or 21 days. If you fast before each season, you will prevent getting any of the illnesses that that particular season brings. Fasting helps prevent your body from being off balance. This is especially true during the Spring season. If we fast right before and up until the first of Spring, we will be showered with abundance, health, wealth, joy and inner peace. Spring is also a good time to begin new projects. Cleansing during this time will assure success in the project. Spring is the time for renewal, cleansing, beauty and coming out. Be in tune and receive your divine gifts.

During menstruation: Women should fast two days before the onset of their menstrual flow and all during their menstruation to prevent or minimize pre-menstrual syndrome (PMS), headaches, pain, heavy bleeding and clotting, mood swings and nausea.

Fast to unblock / to clear the way: If you are experiencing blockages in your life in the form of lack of money flow, in relationships, on your job, in your profession, in your heart or your health, then fast and purify to clear any lack or limitation.

The How of Nutritional Fasting

Queen Afua is the originator of the 21-Day Urban City Group Fast and the 21-Day New Year's Fast. Her fasting method has been used by several other centers throughout the New York metropolitan area.

The 21-Day Fast

For advanced students of fasting the 21-Day Fast is very effective, particularly to do so as the seasons change or to effect major changes in your life quickly. This is what you can expect for each week of your 21 days.

First week (Degree 1, 1-7 days): Elimination of old waste, a rapid clearing within the physical body. This week is when you must pull on your strength to get through the first 3-4 days of fasting. These days separate the weak from the strong. If you pass these days, you have pretty much no problem thereafter. The "fastens crisis" usually occurs during the first 3-4 days. Follow the instructions included in this book as to what to do during the crisis in order to come out of it as quickly as possible.

Second week (Degree 2, 8-14 days): This week you become physically stronger than ever before. You have more endurance; your body becomes more flexible because the poisons are coming out of the joints. You are able to do things with your body temple that you did 5-10 years ago. You can walk faster, and have less problems walking up stairs. Your breathing will be deeper and fuller. Your mind is sharper and more creative. Your skin will glow. That book or proposal that you were trying to write previously is now being written effortlessly. We think we might have less energy when we fast. If you use this method of cleansing and rejuvenating, you will have more energy with each given day that you fast.

Third week (Degree 3, 15-21 days): This is the week when you open up spiritually, when you can hear that still, small voice of the Most High Allah, Almighty God. You are now in your divine state, like that of a holy wo/man. You are more peaceful, relaxed, slow to anger, if at all, more tolerant of others, stress-less and joyous. You smile and laugh more now and you can see the beauty of life. Others will look up to you and ask guidance in the affairs for the light of wisdom, spiritual beauty and peace is flowing from you. Your aches and pains are gone physically, spiritually and emotionally. Repeat the 21 days often if you desire to maintain a high state in an impure world. Fasting is a

way for you to truly become "high." Taking drugs and
alcohol is not getting you high, it's taking you low. If we
all fasted throughout the world, crime, violence and war
would be eliminated on the planet Earth.

Once you come off a long fast, eat only fruits and
vegetables for 14 days. If you come off the fast and begin
eating even whole grains and vegetable proteins or meat,
you will reverse the benefits of the fast and get sick. So eat
light foods, continue drinking your juices and stay in
peacefulness.

Alternating the Nutritional Fasting and Natural Living
method of diet is an excellent lifestyle. It provides for body
cleansing with little or no residual stress or strain. You
can fast and rejuvenate in this manner without supervision.

When embarking on the 21-Day Fasting Program, it is
advised that you seek supervision from a knowledgeable
person experienced in guiding you through this longer
fasting process.

With each fast you do you are constantly spiraling up
the pyramid toward the top of consciousness, never to
return to the land of darkness. You are constantly moving
toward more light, brilliance, clarity, power and peace.

Talk Fast

For a period of time daily for spiritual strengthening,
particularly during a fast, one should avoid talking for 1-2
hours. This is called your *hour of power*. This process
develops meditation opportunities. Once you peacefully
close the portals called the lips, the other portals of
communication become more activated, such as the "third
eye" and crown chakras. From these centers you are able
to "hear" the Holy Spirit talk through and to you. When
these chakras are open, you receive inner spiritual
guidance in your daily affairs. This exercise also helps to
detoxify your thoughts and release adverse thought
processes. It then allows for your mind to experience
higher thoughts and visions.

Fasting For World Peace and Health
No more internal or external wars;
there is hope, but we must fast and pray.

Families: Guide your family members to do consistent fasting together and watch the love build in the family unit. Teachers: Take your students through a 3-7 day fast or live food diet weekly. Watch the improvement in your students' performance.

P.T.A. Members: Fast for 2 days before each meeting and see how smoothly the meeting goes and how much work is accomplished.

CEOs: Have your company members fasted for 24 hours to 3-7 days each month? If so, have you observed that less sick leave time is taken, there is greater cooperation among staff and sales increase. Employees will be happier on the job because the atmosphere will be so pleasant. Fasting is cost effective for the company. Hire a fasting expert to motivate and guide your staff weekly and monthly.

Unions: Ms. Anna Mae Massey, Chairwoman of the Health Committee under the leadership of Mr. Al Diop, President of the largest municipal labor union #1549 DC37, as keynote speaker was able to inform and inspire approximately 200 members of the value of fasting and cleansing. These union members went on a weekend health retreat. They ate light, healthy foods, drank fresh juices, received healing massages and attended workshops on stress management, holistic health, nutrition, food alternatives and exercise. The participants felt love and gave love that weekend. More unions and businesses need to follow this format.

Presidents, National and Civic Leaders: You should fast every seasonal change for 7-21 days and 24 hours weekly. Decisions made for a country would become the highest decision for the greater good. A president should encourage citizens to fast 24 hours weekly or 1 to 3 days a month for unity and purity. They should fast to fight crime and bring peace throughout the land. Gandhi fasted to give his people freedom. When the people are pure, there is peace.

The violence in the cities and in the land is greatly due to "fast foods" (causing fast death). High sugar intake is causing over-reaction, hyperactivity and mental depression. Eating meat causes people to become more violent and animalistic in nature.

Heads of State: Prior to convening the General Assembly of the United Nations, the representatives should fast for 3 days. This would help prepare them for their tasks of holding peace talks and making decisions that affect the world.

Ministers, Imams, Priests, Rabbis and all religious leaders: You should fast 1-3 days weekly or 7 days a month to live totally on the Holy Word and to be a living example of purity in body, mind and spirit. The cleansing of the leaders will increase the number of followers on particular spiritual paths. There will be more light, love and wisdom coming from the spiritual leader when s/he is living as the ancients by — "fasting and prayer." Spiritual leaders should encourage their congregations to fast on holy days, to eat only spiritual food on those days (not the food of the earth) so that before and after the service they will be living and breathing the Spirit. Also, if consistent fasting is encouraged, there will be little or no sickness amongst the followers. No more high blood pressure, weight problems, asthma, premature aging, etc. The members will receive healing spiritually and physically by the example of their leaders' guidance and lifestyles. "Be ye perfect" and purified.

Purification and Rejuvenation as a Way of Life

A wonderful, fantastic, ecstatic, fulfilling way of living. A gift supreme. Explosive! Oh so powerful! Makes you feel clean on the inside. Look beautiful on the outside. Embrace your healing; digest it; caress it; fall back on it; move forward with it; stand on it; lean on it; rest on it. It will build you into a perfect temple of pure light, love, wealth and health.

Combining the Nutritional Fasting and Natural Living programs harmonizes the body, mind and spirit. The body, mind and spirit grow and develop collectively and in unison. As you rise and graduate to higher levels in your fasting and natural living, you will bear witness to your heightened spiritual and mental progression. As you work through these various levels observe how fear, anger, depression, anxiety, lack of faith fall from you. Observe instead that with each step of purification you advance toward perfection. Observe a greater capacity for love, peace, faith, humility, wealth and health radiate through around and about you.

On the mind: The Creator will live in your mind and thoughts. You will gain greater intelligence and creativity that is boundless and unlimited.

On physical wealth: You will become more prosperous. Our Mother Father God has many mansions. Because you are the sons and daughters of a great Creator, you are the heirs and heiresses to the throne. If you will but allow the Divine Holy Spirit to guide you and keep you in your business affairs, you shall be triumphant. As you move with joy and great expectation through these high degrees of purification and rejuvenation, your whole world opens like that of a thousand petal lotus. All is contained in the crown chakra of your being. Once purified, your centers can be activated and you can become pure light and love. As you continue to cleanse your body temple, that still, quiet inner voice is able to guide you so that you may be victorious in all your affairs. So go on and grow through freshmen, sophomore, junior and senior levels. Become like Methuselah, who lived to be 976 years of age, and the other ancients who lived for hundreds of years because they were in harmony in body, mind and spirit.

Chapter 6

BEFORE YOU BEGIN

It is suggested that you read this entire section before beginning your two-cycle cleansing. It is especially important to read *Detoxification, Questions,* and *Breaking the Nutritional Fast.*

Detoxification

Dare to be Great! Purify! Once you start fasting (i.e., living off of fruit and vegetable juices) your body will begin to detoxify, getting rid of wastes and poisons that have been in your body for years. All fasters experience cleansing reactions at the onset of their fast. First of all, don't be alarmed for it is a natural reaction and is to be expected. You may experience anywhere from one to three different cleansing reactions. The more preparation you put into starting the fast (eating more raw fruits and vegetables), the less you may experience the "faster's detox." Here's a list of some of the things you may experience during the first few days of fasting.

Fasting or Cleansing Crises

Headaches	Nightmares Dizziness	Shortness of breath
Skin eruptions		Flatulence/passing gas
Weakness	Mental confusion	Heavy Breathing
No patience	Blurred Vision	High blood pressure
Tiredness	Depression	Fevers
Aches and pains	Vaginal discharge	Mood Swings

These reactions come from a history of poor diet, nighttime eating, too much starch, too much sugar and heavy meat intake, along with consuming excessive fried foods and dairy products. The reactions you may experience can last from one hour to two or three years.

☞ The best way to help your body adjust to these changes is to first discontinue taking all fruit juices until the symptoms subside. Continue taking your vegetable juice combinations. Taking only vegetable juices will stabilize and strengthen the body before deeper cleansing can continue by taking fruit juices. *Note: Juice combinations will be given later.*

☞ Take low enemas immediately, using only warm water in a quart size enema bag. Discontinue taking salt baths for two days. Take warm showers instead. Give yourself a vigorous massage starting at your foot and working upwards toward your heart. You may even want to have a professional massage.

☞ Discontinue taking your kidney-liver flush. Replace it with the juice of one lemon, three tablespoons of cold-pressed olive oil and eight ounces of warm water. Also drink a mixture of dandelion and alfalfa tea. (Use two teaspoons of each herb in two cups of water. Steep for two hours.) Get more rest and sleep.

If you follow these instructions, your cleansing reactions should be over within one to three days. If the symptoms persist, please contact your fasting consultant or get an emergency colon cleansing. Some fasters who were on a light vegetarian diet before fasting usually found that they did not experience any of the reactions listed earlier.

One key thing to remember throughout fasting is to constantly give yourself intense prayer treatments. Call on your God for your restoration and healing with your heart and soul. If you cleanse and rejuvenate regularly and consistently, you can expect to rid the body of all the diseases that were mentioned earlier, as well as eliminating all other chronic diseases, such as: *High blood pressure; Arthritis; Asthma, Hay fever and allergies; Female disorders (cysts, tumors, heavy menstruation); Prostrate gland disorders.*
Note: For heavy bleeding, take Shepherd's purse and comfrey.

Commonly asked Questions about the Natural Living and Nutritional Fasting Process

1) *How do I get my nutrients (minerals and vitamins) during the fast?*
A: Your nutrients are in the spirulina, herbs and juices you will take.

2) *Will I have enough energy during the fast?*
A: If you eat light (fruits, vegetables and water) for 1 week or more before a fast and take at least 1-2 enemas or herbal laxatives, you will be on "high" throughout the fast. If not, increase your spirulina or *Heal Thyself Nutritional Formula* to an additional teaspoon with juice and take an additional enema for greater energy.

3) *Can I go to work while fasting?*
A: By all means! The Urban City Fast, the original name of my Nutritional Fasting method, is designed to allow you to live as much of a "normal" life as possible. If you prepare 1-2 weeks for your fast, you should have no problems while working. During your work hours, your fasting should be a pleasant experience.

4) *How do I handle social engagements, holidays and going out to restaurants?*
A: Invite your friends or business associates out to a vegetarian restaurant. Learn the various food alternatives and follow some of the recipes within this book. There are prepared meat substitutes in most health food stores, or you may prefer to prepare your meat alternatives in your own kitchen.

5) *Will I feel deprived?*
A: View your cleansing as a gift that you are giving to yourself, the "Gift of Life." See the rejuvenation process as a fun and exciting journey or like the beautiful lotus opening up within you. Follow the "Food Alternative List" that is within this book. You

are not going to be able to eat many of the foods you
are used to eating. However, the alternatives are
healthier.

6) *What if people make fun of me?*
A: Take the path of least resistance. Laugh with them,
then share your tabouli and okra, tofu dip with
seaweed crackers, freshly prepared pear juice or
banana ice cream. You may have a convert.

7) *Suppose my spouse thinks I'm crazy?*
A: Prepare a natural bubble bath and add rose petals to
the water. Put on soft music as you welcome your
spouse in a bath fit for a king or queen. Massage your
spouse's feet with almond oil. While your spouse is in
a tub, serve fresh pressed fruit juice in a long-
stemmed glass. Do this just as s/he emerges from the
bath. Have a freshly prepared salad, steamed vegetables with a vegetarian protein or baked fish waiting.
Put a candle and flowers on a table. Your spouse will
no longer think you are crazy. S/he will love the
change in you since you started the path of purification and will probably join you on it.

8) *Is it necessary to take a daily enema?*
A: Yes. Your body is releasing toxins daily. An enema
will ease the burden that the body is going through in
trying to eliminate the waste. Your colon is in a state
of rest while you are fasting so you will be not
eliminating as much waste on your own. As a result,
if poisons that have not loosened are left unattended
in the body, the body will feed off its own waste. You
will then experience headaches, anger, dizziness,
blurred vision, etc. Taking daily enemas will ward off
these symptoms.

9) *What is a colonic?*
A: A colonic is a form of hydrotherapy. It is a deep
cleansing of the colon. Between 5-15 gallons of water

flow in and out (through) your colon carrying out old impacted waste, gas and toxins.

10) *I experienced a headache during the first several days. Why and what can I do to stop it?*
A: You are experiencing a "faster's crisis." Take enemas immediately. Discontinue drinking fruit juices for 24 to 36 hours. To stabilize yourself drink only vegetable juices. Discontinue the kidney-liver flush. Just drink lemon juice and water for your breakfast. Take only showers during this time. No salt baths. In addition, rest as much as you can.

11) *Why is it important to take epsom salt baths?*
A: The salt and water is like that of an ocean bath. It helps to relax the body and release stress. It also draws poisons out through the pores.

12) *I felt dizzy while in the bath. Why and what can I do about it?*
A: You are eliminating toxins from poisonous foods and drugs taken into your system. If you feel dizzy, decrease your salt bath from 4 to 2 pounds. By the next bath, try to use 3 to 4 pounds of salt. If your diet has been light, you'll be able to take more salt.

13) *What if I stray?*
A: Don't put yourself down in any way. Love, support and nurture yourself throughout your healing process. It takes time to grow.
    Take an enema or herbal laxative, healing bath or vegetable juices immediately. These forms of natural healing will put you back on track and in harmony in yourself. The more you actively do the correct things the less likely you are to stray.

14) *How do you know when you are ready to go to the next level?*
A: You will no longer crave for particular foods. That is, you will begin to eat fewer foods and desire to drink

more fresh juices and eat more salads. The more you cleanse, take enemas, herbal laxatives, drink vegetable juices, the less you will desire heavy foods.

15. *Should I discontinue taking my medication when I begin your fast or any other?*
A: Do not discontinue taking your medication without your doctor's consent. As you use natural food, herbs and juices to rejuvenate your body, your doctor will see an improvement in your health and lessen the quantity of medication or will even remove you from it altogether. Have patience. Returning your system back to a state of total health takes time.

Some of these questions were formulated by my friend lawyer and devotee of purification, Dianne Ciccone, and Marcia Lily, a devotee of purification for over nine years. I thank them dearly for being in tune with the heartbeat of the people, to know what questions needed answers.

Chapter 7

Natural Living: Cycles I & II with Juice Recommendations

Rejuvenation + Purification = Harmony in Body, Mind and Spirit

Rejuvenation = Vegetables (live and steamed), chlorophyll, wheatgrass and spirulina; rejuvenating herbs.

Purification = Enemas, herbal laxatives and colonics; purification herbs; fruits.

Levels of Mastery

Freshman — Organically-fed chicken and fish (unshelled fish) baked or broiled; 75% steamed vegetables, 25% raw vegetables.
Whole grains — brown rice, bulgar wheat.

Sophomore — Soya meats, beans, peas, nuts, seeds and sprouts.
50% steamed-, 50% raw-vegetables.
Whole grains — brown rice, burger wheat.

Junior — Sprouts (alfalfa, mung and others).
25% steamed-, 75% raw-vegetables.
Light grains such as tabouli and couscous.

Senior — Live uncooked foods and sprouted proteins.
100% raw diet of fresh fruits, vegetables, juices; nuts and seeds (eaten in moderation).

Master — 50% of diet — juices and herd teas.
50% of diet — fresh fruits and vegetables
No grains, nuts or seeds.

Ph.d.   A "Ph.d." purified diet would consist of
                100% pure air and pure water. Alas, we
                must first cleanse the planet.

Cycle I: Natural Living Diet
(Alternate with the Nutritional Fasting Diet as a natural lifestyle.)

Pre-breakfast: Juice of one lemon with 8 oz. warm water.
                Up to 2 tbsp. of cold-pressed olive oil with
                drops of Kyolic or 2 tbsp. of the Colon
                Deblocker. (*This is to be taken two times a week
                only*).

The pre-breakfast is to be taken upon first rising, and
at least 30 minutes before eating or drinking or anything
else. Its purpose is to enhance the cleansing process that
the body experiences during sleep. The lemon juice helps
to remove mucus. The cold-pressed olive oil lubricates the
colon and facilitates elimination. The garlic, or Kyolic (an
odorless garlic extract) cleanses the blood and the cayenne
(not recommended in cases of high blood pressure)
improves circulation.

Breakfast: Vegetable and fruit juice
                1 tbsp. Queen Afua's Super Nutritional
                Formula
                1-2 pieces of fruit

Breakfast consists of 2 to 3 servings of fresh fruit, such
as grapefruits, oranges, papaya, pear, ½ pound of grapes,
melons, particularly watermelons, plums, mangoes,
cherries. If you eat bananas, they should be well ripened
with plenty of spots. Try to concentrate on fruits that have
been specially recommended to you. Don't eat dried fruits
because of the concentrated sugar that will destroy your
teeth. After eating all fruit, brush with Queen Afua's Clay
and a non-abrasive toothbrush.

Lunch: Large raw salad with plenty sprouts. All sorts
                of green leafy vegetables; do not steam for more
                than 3-4 minutes.

For your protein source eat lentils, peas, sprouts, tofu or soya meats. Beans must be soaked over-night. However, do not eat more than 2 oz. of nuts or seeds. No peanuts or cashew nuts.

If you are not a vegetarian, you may eat baked or broiled unshelled fish no more than 1 or 2 times weekly. No shellfish (lobster, clams, or shrimp). Try to follow this only as a transitional diet until you become a vegetarian.

Add 1 tbsp. of Heal Thyself Super Nutritional Formula with juice.

Lunch should comprise a large salad, steamed leafy greens and a protein. The salad is made of raw vegetables (try to include plenty of okra) with a light salad dressing. *No mayonnaise or other dairy products, please!* Green leafy vegetables (kale, dandelion; mustard) can be steamed 4-5 minutes.

You should eliminate all animal products (beef, chicken, fish, milk and other dairy products). You will get your proteins from lentils, peas, tofu, sprouts, and meat substitutes that are not made from eggs.

If you are going to eat starches like couscous, millet, brown rice, then eat them with vegetables for better digestion.

One or more vegetable juice combinations has been recommended to cleanse and strengthen the body. This should be made with a vegetable juicer (not a blender) and consumed immediately after juicing for greater healing properties to be present.

Dinner: Repeat lunch meal.
           No protein or starch after 7 p.m.
           1 tbsp. Super Nutritional Formula with juice.

Dinner is a repetition of lunch. All cooked food should be eaten before the sun goes down. Afterwards, eat live foods (raw fruits and vegetables). Drink a pint to one quart of distilled or purified water.

Cycle II: Nutritional Fasting
Purification for Liberation

Degree I Beginning students	75% vegetable juice, 25% fruit juice.
Degree II Intermediate students	50% vegetable juice, 50% fruit juice.
Degree III Advanced students	Fruit juices
	Wheatgrass 4 oz. or more
	Spirulina, 2-3 tablespoons three times a day in 1 quart to 1 gallon of water.

It took me 16 years to master a natural living and fasting as a way of life and diet. It is a process. Be sure to read how to begin and how to come off nutritional fasts in the *Fasting* section of this book. Above all, be consistent and patient.

Cycle II: Nutritional Fasting Diet
(Alternate with Seven Day Natural Living Diet as a natural lifestyle.)

<u>Pre-breakfast:</u>	Kidney-liver flush: juice of 1 lemon, 3 tbsp. Colon Deblocker, 12 drops of liquid Kyolic, 1 pinch to ¼ teaspoon cayenne pepper and 8 oz. distilled water.
<u>Breakfast:</u>	Fruit juice (8-12 oz.)
<u>Lunch:</u>	Vegetable juice (8-12 oz.)
	(Vegetable juice must be prepared fresh for greatest potency. If you can't obtain fresh juice at lunch time, then drink fruit juice now and prepare the fresh vegetable juice for breakfast.)
<u>Dinner:</u>	Vegetable juice (12-16 oz.)
<u>Nutrients:</u>	Take 1 tbsp. of Super Nutritional Formula with each juice meal.

A word to the wise: If you must prepare dinner for your loved ones while fasting, be sure to drink 12 oz. of vegetable juice with your nutrients before you begin preparing the meal to eliminate any desire to taste the food you are preparing. Drink at least 6-8 glasses of pure water daily.

During Cycles I and II, your daily and weekly routines should include: internal cleansing (nasal and colon), bathing, physical exercise and activity, drinking Master Herbal formulas, clay applications and spiritual mediation or prayer.
(See the following pages and appropriate sections in this book for further instructions on the above.)

Internal cleansing	Enemas should be taken daily while on the fast. Add the juice of one lemon to the water. (Also see the *Hydrotherapy* chapter.)
External cleansing	Baths — Use 4 drops Eucalyptus oil, and/or 4 lbs. Epsom salt in a tub of warm water. (***Note:*** *Salt should not be used if you have high blood pressure. Use herbs and oils instead.*) Take 3 times a week. Soak body for 30 min. Massage body in an upward motion toward heart while in tub. Take a shower after bath. (Also see chapter on *Hydrotherapy*.)
Clay application	For major problems, use a clay pack with gauze overnight. For minor problems, use during day and evening hours.
Physical activity	See *Chapter 16* of this book.
Tonics	Take the Master Herbal Formula 4-7 times a week. Preparation: boil 4-5 cups of water; turn off flame; add 3 teaspoons of herbs to water and steep overnight. Drink in the morning.

JUICE RECOMMENDATIONS
Drink Juices every day for Cleansing and Rejuvenation!

Vegetable Juice Combinations

Carrot/beet   For blood cleansing and building ¼, ½
or 1 whole beet and 1 or more carrots.
Take small amounts in the beginning to
avoid a fasting "detox" reaction.
*Note: Don't use beets if you have high
blood pressure.*

Cucumber,   For édema; to relieve water retention
carrot, parsley and aid in kidney healing.
1 or more carrots, ½ to 1 whole
cucumber (remove skin, if waxed)
and ½ bunch of parsley.

Carrot/celery   For relaxation (anti-stress)
2 stalks of celery and 1 or more carrots.
*Note: Don't use celery if you have high
blood pressure due to high sodium con-
tent.*

Carrot/scallion To clear congestion from lungs.
1-2 radishes, 1 or more carrots and 1
teaspoon horseradish.

Carrot/ginger   To increase circulation
1 or more carrots with ¼ cup of freshly
pressed ginger.

Carrot/leek   To eliminate high blood pressure.
3 or more carrots and 1-2 pieces of leek.

Carrot/turnip   To relieve arthritis in joints: 3 or more
carrots with 1 turnip. *This is a bone
knitter*

Carrot/cabbage For indigestion: 3 or more carrots with a

quarter of a cabbage.

String beans and carrots	For diabetes: 1 or more carrots and ½ lb. string beans.
Pure green drink	For body restoration ½-1 whole bunch of parsley, a few sprigs of watercress, 2-3 leaves of kale and ½ of a cucumber.

Fruit Juice Combinations

Apple	Helps cleanse the blood. It acts as a natural laxative.
Pineapple	Fights congestion and helps remove mucus.
Cranberry	Helps fight cancer and cleanses the blood.
Papaya	Helps relieve indigestion.
Grapefruit, orange/lemon	Helps to eliminate respiratory difficulties, sinus congestion and vaginal discharges.
Grape	Helps cleanse the blood and aids the elimination of mucus forming food residue.

According to the "Juice Man," wash fruits and vegetables with the juice of one lemon, a few teaspoons of sea salt (dissolved in a quart of pure water). Or according to *Heal Thyself*, use 2 tablespoons of Dr. Bronner's liquid soap diluted in 1-2 quarts of pure water. Be sure to rinse the fruits and vegetables with pure water.

For foods that have been waxed, such as apples and cucumbers, cut off the skin before juicing. Better yet, use organic fruits and vegetables, i.e. grown without the use of poisonous sprays.

Chapter 8

Life After Nutritional Fasting

When you are coming off a 21-Day Fast, or for that matter a 7-day fast, the return to solid foods must be done gradually. Some of your old eating patterns and habits will change according to how often you fast and cleanse. Be prepared to give up heavy foods as you progress with each cleansing.

It takes 2-4 weeks to come off the fast properly. Avoid eating too much, too heavy or too late in the evening in order to avoid getting sick or being constipated in the morning. If you break your fast too quickly, you may experience nausea, dizziness, depression or anger. You may even re-gain the weight you lost, swell up, get tired, or experience aches and pains. If you return to your old diet, your diseases will also return. Use your fasting as a stepping stone for moving away from over-processed, hard to digest foods such as meats, fried foods, sugar, dairy and "junk food."

Incorporate these additional points in your normal health maintenance program after any fast.

- Take vegetable juice 1-2 times daily.
- Take nutrients 2 twice daily.
- Take 2 enemas weekly.
- Allow yourself 15 minutes of exercise daily.
- Take salt baths 3 times a week.
- Continue clay packs until problem has cleared up.

Breaking a 7-Day Fast

Day 1   Eat only vegetables, raw or steamed.

Day 2   Include fruits to diet.

Days 3-6   Include vegetarian proteins. For meat eaters, include baked fish and whole grains, but eat only in very small portions.

(One protein or starch for the day could include sprouts, tofu, beans, peas and lentils.)

Day 7   Discontinue starches and all proteins except sprouts, particularly if you follow the lifestyle of 7 days of fasting and 7 days of the Natural Living Diet. Eat light on the 7th day and take an enema or herbal laxative to prepare you for your 7 days of fasting so that you won't experience a toxic reaction while on the fast.

Breaking a 21-Day Fast

1st week   Days 1-2: Eat vegetables; steam them for 3-4 minutes. Also eat a vegetable salad. Consume as much okra as possible for it has a natural laxative effect.
Days 3-7: Include fruits. Eat a grapefruit each day. Do not eat bananas until two weeks after the fast is over. When you do, make sure the bananas are well spotted as they will be in a state that is easier to digest.

2nd week   Include small portions of vegetarian protein, such as lentils, peas, beans (soak overnight and prepare with ginger or bay leaf for better digestion), sprouts, eggless soymeats or miso soup. Eat plenty of vegetables, raw and steamed, with proteins.

3rd week   Include whole grain starches, such as couscous, millet, bulgar wheat, tabouli, brown rice, sprouted whole grain toasted bread.

4th week   If you have a great desire to eat flesh, eat unshelled baked fish. No chicken, beef, pork or lamb. Avoid all dairy products from cows or goats such as milk, cheese and ice cream. Use soya milk and tofutti as a calcium source instead. Also, eat green leafy vegetables and drink oatstraw, comfrey and alfalfa herb teas.

I've found that it takes a season to heal. Generally we begin to study at the onset of a season, for instance, from September to December or January to April. Through many years of observation I've found that it takes a season of uninterrupted self-healing to truly "Heal Thyself." For the serious student of healing, I recommend the pyramid program of self-transformation.

If after you have successfully completed this program season you decide to return to low vibration poisonous foods, your body will react by detoxing immediately in the form of a runny nose, coughing, headaches, dizziness, pain, rage or depression. You have outgrown lower levels of food consumption. The toxic reaction indicates that you have risen to higher levels of your health. You have a great deal of light and vitality stored up within your body temple. Therefore, you repel disease-forming matter and can no longer participate in lower ways of living. So, if you have reactions from New Year's egg nog, 4th-of-July's fried chicken or the family reunion's sweet potato pies and collard greens stewed in lard, "run for your life" to the hydrotherapy room (bathroom) in your home. Hurry! Take an enema and healing bath so that you may return swiftly to your natural state of total health. As you purge from deep within your being, "bless your diseases away."

Non-Stop Uninterrupted
Natural Healing for Success

Within every two week cycle, your body temple will progressively build upon itself. By the time you reach the 1000 Lotus Petal, Crown Chakra or Divine Wisdom Center located at the top of your pyramid, complete healing will be accomplished. You alternate for 12 weeks beginning with 7 days of Natural Living followed by 7 days of Nutritional Fasting. Study and follow the instructions given in this chapter as your guide.

Once you've reached the ultimate destination, place a gold star at the top of your *Body Temple Three Month Pyramid Chart.*

In accomplishing this three month self-healing process you will be liberated from addictive poisonous foods, drink and smoke. You will then be able to accept freely the 7/7 *system* as away of life.

Food is your medication — *Eat to live; don't live to eat.*

Note: This program does not diagnose or prescribe. If under a doctor's supervision please continue with medication.

Human Pyramid Power
Every Step Goes Higher and Higher!
Three Months to Create a New You!

1. The pyramid represents: Enlightenment, Resurrection, Divinity, Wisdom and Illumination. As you step higher up the pyramid ladder you become one of "the Shining Ones," — Peaceful, Pure, Powerful and Potent.
2. Use the 7/7 *Three Month Pyramid Program* on the onset of the seasons, Spring, Summer, Fall and Winter.
3. When the body is in an open stance, it takes on the form of the pyramid. The pyramid is a form that is used as a healing symbol of humankind striving toward perfection.
4. As you raise and energize your healing awareness,

the Crown Chakra (energy center) awakens and then you are fully purified (healed) and spiritually realized (enlightened).

5. It will take 84 steps (days) to reach Cosmic Consciousness, which is 75-100% self-healing according to the Heal Thyself Method illustrated in this chart.

6. Six cycles (which is 12 weeks) gives you enough time to maximize and actualize your physical, spiritual, as well as business and romantic goals.

Human Pyramid of Power Chart
Three Month 7/7 Chart for Resurrection of Body, Mind and Spirit

Heru — the Divine Spirit within You

100% Healing = Enlightenment

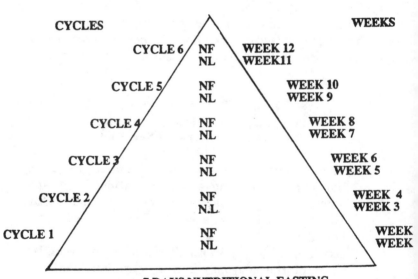

CYCLES		WEEKS
CYCLE 6	NF / NL	WEEK 12 / WEEK11
CYCLE 5	NF / NL	WEEK 10 / WEEK 9
CYCLE 4	NF / NL	WEEK 8 / WEEK 7
CYCLE 3	NF / NL	WEEK 6 / WEEK 5
CYCLE 2	NF / N.L.	WEEK 4 / WEEK 3
CYCLE 1	NF / NL	WEEK / WEEK

7 DAYS NUTRITIONAL FASTING
7 DAYS NATURAL LIVING

Code: Natural Living = NL (pure foods)
Nutritional Fasting = NF Juice fast)
Every 7 days you alternate between NL & NF.

Nutrition and Alternative Foods

As is indicated throughout this book, the food we eat can either become our poison or our medicine. This list indicates the foods which you should avoid and which ones are preferable. Meat, dairy, processed foods and sugar cause most of the health problems that people experience. Removing them from your diet will improve your health, energy level, mood, and mental clarity. It may take a while to make all of the necessary adjustments, but you will see a noticeable improvement. For each of the foods on the low vibration list that you eliminate you will find yourself closer to a disease-free, healthy, youthful and powerful body.

Low Vibration Food (Foods to eliminate)	High Vibration Food (Recommended vital foods)
Cow's milk	Soy-, nut-, goat-, human-milk; kefir
Ice cream	Soy ice cream, tofutti
Cheese	Rennetless unsalted cheese or grated tofu
Margarine	Soya margarine
Yogurt	Brown Cow yogurt*
Eggs	Organic eggs*
White bread	Whole wheat and cracked wheat bread (toasted bread)
Vinegar	Organic apple cider vinegar
Salt	Sea salt, kelp, dulse
Chocolate	Carob
Gelatin	Agar-agar (use to make "Jello" with your favorite fruit juice)
Water	Distilled or spring water
Bottle/can fruit juice	Fresh squeezed/pressed fruit juice
Grocery peanut butter	Fresh unsweetened peanut butter
Junk food	Freshly prepared popcorn, brown rice cakes, dried fruits (such as banana chips, pineapple, apricots, raisins), banana custard, frozen juice (instead of ices), chilled fruit, baked apples, blue corn chips, seaweed chips, whole wheat pretzels, unsalted potato chips prepared

| | in sesame or olive oil. |
| Shellfish | Unshelled fish (clean and garnish with fresh lemon to eliminate some of the bacteria. Eventually try to eliminate flesh foods altogether. |

* Although these two items are listed as alternatives, try to eventually eliminate these foods as well.

Note: Shellfish includes lobster, shrimp, clams, etc., which are scavengers of the ocean. They eat waste in the ocean. When we eat them we further poison ourselves.

Deep/stir-fried foods (Clog the arteries.)	Steam food. Remove from flame. Add 1-2 tbsp. cold-pressed (uncooked) oil to food
White macaroni	Whole wheat macaroni
White rice	Brown rice
White flour	Whole wheat or barley flour
Other grains	Millet, couscous, bulgar
Pancakes	Buckwheat, whole wheat, bran, flaxseed
Grits	Soy grits, barley grits
Oil	Cold-pressed olive oil
Cornmeal cereal†	Whole oats, granola
Corn starch	Arrowroot powder
White sugar	Raw honey, maple syrup, blackstrap molasses, fructose
Protein: meat, poultry, fish	Sprouts, tofu, miso, seeds (sesame, pumpernickel, sunflower), nuts (pecan, walnut, pistachio, almonds), beans (black, pinto, kidney, etc.), peas (black-eye, etc.) Also use soya meats as an alternative.
Canned/frozen vegetables	Fresh vegetables (steamed or raw)
Soda	Fresh juice, mineral water or Perrier water

† i.e., corn flakes or "sugar pops"

In the place of dairy (milk, cheese, ice cream), eat soya products.

Note: Eat whole grain starches only three times a week during the hours of 12-4 p.m., or not at all.

Natural Vitamin Supplements

Calcium	Oatstraw and comfrey herbs, sprouts, carrots, green leafy vegetables, nutmilk and soya milk
Vitamin A & D	Carrots
Vitamin B	Yeast and bee pollen
Vitamin C	Rosehips herb tea
Vitamin E	Alfalfa, wheatgrass
Minerals	Kelp, other sea plants such as spirulina and blue-green manna.

Nature has provided us with a great variety of fruits and vegetables, beans and whole grains so that we need never be bored for eating simply and naturally. Remember to use organic, unsprayed fruits and vegetables whenever possible.

Recommended Fruits

Sweet fruits	Pomegranates, bananas, dates, raisins, dried apples and dried apricots
Sub-acid fruits	Mangoes, peaches, plums, pears, green grapes, dark grapes, papaya
Acid fruits	Strawberries, raspberries, blueberries pineapple, grapefruits, oranges, lemons, tomatoes. boysenberries
Melons	Cantaloupes, watermelon, honeydew melon (to be eaten alone)

Recommended Vegetables

Asparagus	Onions	Dandelions
Beets	Okra	Irish potatoes
Celery	Parsley	Lettuce
Cabbage	Greens of all kinds	Swiss chard
Cauliflower	Watercress	All sprouts
Carrots	Parsnip	Spinach
Cucumbers	Pumpkin	Beans
Turnips	Rutabagas	Squash
Tomatoes	Sweet potatoes	

Starches	Millet, tabouli, couscous, corn-on-the-cob, pumpkin, bulgur wheat, squash, coconut, potato, yam.
Seaweed	Dulse, nori, hijiki.
Proteins	String-, green-, wax-, lima-, navy-, kidney-, soy-beans; split peas, lentils, chick peas, pigeon peas.
Sprouts	Alfalfa, mung.
Nuts and Seeds	Almonds, walnuts, filberts, brazil, pecans, sunflower, sesame and pumpkin seeds.

Avoid Mucus-forming Foods

Mucus forming foods contribute to many poor health conditions, such as colds, shortness of breath, fevers, hay fever, asthma, loss of hearing and sight, constipation, female disorders (such as tumors, cysts, vaginal discharge, PMS) male prostrate gland blockage, fatigue, weight problems and mental congestion.

To eliminate excess and unhealthy mucus from your body temple, in the mornings drink freshly prepared juice of 2 grapefruits, 2 oranges and ½ lemon or the freshly prepared pineapple juice. Dilute either by ½ with water.

In the mornings you will expel mucus from nose, eyes, ears, vagina (if a woman) and anus. The more mucus that comes out of the body, the closer you are to returning to a disease-free body.

To support your cleansing further, take 2 herbal laxatives weekly until the problem is eliminated. Other methods include: senna and peppermint (1 teaspoon of each herb steeped for 1 hour), powdered aloe (¼ teaspoon in water), cascara sagrada (1 teaspoon in water or 3 capsules), or *Heal Thyself Colon Deblocker* (3 tablespoons with lemon water taken 3 times a week).

Special Meals for the Person in Transition from Meat Eating

On the day you eat one of these meals, take a herbal laxative, eat plenty of okra, or fast the next day on a diet of 50% fruit juices and 50% vegetable juices only.

Meatless Meals for Lunch and Dinner

1) Soya meat (in place of turkey or fish), steamed broccoli with chopped scallions and a garden salad.

2) Baked sweet potatoes, bulgur wheat "meatloaf" (bind with sugarless tomato sauce, onion, peppers and whole wheat flour) and a garden salad.

3) Caribbean meal: Brown rice and peas (this is a poor food combination, but you may have it occasionally), and steamed okra and onions to aid digestion.

4) For picnics, serve barbecue tofu (use a barbecue sauce from a health food store; it should contain no sugar or additives), corn on the cob (use soy margarine and dulse) and Queen Afua's Rainbow Salad.

5) Southern meal: black-eye peas, string beans, whole grain cornmeal corn bread (use any recipe but substitute honey for sugar, egg replacer or agar-agar instead of eggs, soy milk instead of cow's milk). *Note:* Include soaked flaxseed or a few tablespoons of bran to act as a laxative.

Chapter 9

Recipes from Queen Afua's Kitchen Laboratory

Food is our Medicine

Rainbow Salad

½ shredded green cabbage
½ shredded purple cabbage
3 shredded carrots (for calcium, and vitamins A & D)
1 shredded beet (cleanses and builds the blood)
Garnish with parsley around the salad

*Cabbage aids digestion; juice or eat raw.

☞ Mix together with egg-less mayonnaise from your neighborhood food cooperative or health food store and 3 tablespoons of soy sauce.
Do not use soy sauce if you have high blood pressure.

Garden Green Salad

*1 head of lettuce**
1 bunch spinach (for iron)
1 whole red pepper (for vitamin C)
1-2 cups of alfalfa sprouts (a vegetable protein)
½ bunch of watercress
Sprinkle ½ cup of soaked sunflower seeds (optional)

*Do not use Bibb lettuce, for according to the late herbalist, Dr. John Moore, it contains morphine.

☞ Combine ingredients and serve with following dressing: Cold-pressed olive oil (a colon lubricant) and apple cider vinegar (which breaks up mucus and congestion).

High Protein Nut Milk (Shake)

½ cup pumpkin seeds†
3-4 tbsp. tahini butter
1 ripe banana
Maple syrup or blackstrap molasses (for iron)
1 tbsp. lecithin (brain food)

† for restoration of male reproductive organs

☞ Combine in blender. Drink and enjoy.
Note: You can also use almonds, brazil nuts, pecans, sunflower seed. Always soak nuts and seeds.

Ginger Drink (for improved circulation)

1 cup of juiced ginger (for digestion and circulation)
3 lemons or limes (for vitamin C and mucus elimination)
Maple syrup or raw honey

☞ Blend 1 quart purified water with ingredients. Heat slightly during winter months or drink at room temperature.

Tofu Egg Rolls without the Eggs

2 cakes of tofu — mash to a cheesy consistency
½ cup miso or 3 tbsp. tamari/soy sauce with ¼ cup water
1 cup sprouts (mung bean or alfalfa)
2-4 grated carrots

☞ Pour off any liquid after you've blended the ingredients. Lay flat 3-4 sheets of Nori seaweed on wooden board. Put in ½ cup of mixture on the sheet and roll together in the shape of an egg roll. Slice in half.

Tofu on a Bed of Tabouli

Tabouli is a light and easy to digest grain that does not require cooking, thus it produces very little mucus formation or congestion in the body. It's low in calories.

Soak 2 cups tabouli in ½-1 cup
of warm water for 15-20 minutes
Add chopped scallions
1 whole onion
⅓ cup steamed okra†
2 tbsps. sage*

*Don't use sage if breast-feeding. It dries up the milk.
† For a laxative effect which will "sweep out" the system in a few hours)

☞ Add other herbal seasonings that you so desire. Once prepared, place Tabouli on a plate or platter.
   Dice 1 cake of Tofu (a high protein soybean curd) with your desired seasonings in the center of the Tabouli platter.
   Garnish around the Tabouli with parsley (high in iron) to be eaten with this dish.

Tofu Pizza

Pizza Spread — grated tofu, natural tomato sauce (without sugar) or blend 2 tomatoes and 2 teaspoons Italian seasonings

☞ Put a little soya margarine on sprouted whole grain bread and then use Tofu pizza spread.
   Eat a large side order of kale, spinach, okra, or broccoli with any and all starch meals.

Berry Fruit Salad

2 cups of strawberries — sliced in half
1 cup of blueberries
1 cup raspberries
½ cup grated raw coconut
Garnish with 1 cup of chopped pecans

This salad is excellent to cleansing the blood.

Summer Melon Salad

½ watermelon
2 whole cantaloupes
1 whole honeydew melon

☞ Scoop out watermelon first to use as a "boat" for the
fruit of all the melons. Use a melon bail scoop to create
a nice look for the salad.

This salad cleanses the water in your system and
purifies the kidneys. Melons should not be mixed with
any other foods.

Easy Cereal

Couscous and oats as a cereal — to be eaten only 1-2
times a week.

☞ Soak 1 cup of grain in cup of water for 15 mins. If you
cook these grains rather than soak them, you will
become constipated. Add cinnamon, nutmeg or raw
honey as a sweetener.

A half to 1 hour before eating any grain, drink warm
water with lemon or fresh vegetable/fruit juice.

Making your heavy meals light

Whenever you prepare a bean or vegetable bean soup,
add one of the following after the soup has been
completely prepared:

1 cup of diced okra
1 teaspoon of cascara sagrada,
or 1 tablespoon flaxseed (soaked overnight).

This soup 1-2 times a week helps to avoid constipation.

Non-dairy Ice Cream Dessert

☞ Freeze a couple of peeled bananas and 1 cup of strawberries.
Once the above ingredients are frozen, chop up and put
in blender.
Add 2 teaspoons cinnamon or nutmeg, ½ cup walnuts,
and sugarless vanilla (from the health food store).
Add ½-1 cup of water depending on consistency desired.

☞ For ice cream sandwiches, spread the combination over
a rice cake. Sprinkle coconut over the spread and then
place a second rice cake over the coconut. Put in plastic
bags and then in freezer to have ready whenever you
would like a healthy dessert for you and your children.

Bean Soups

Always add vegetables of your choice to your bean
soups. Steep the vegetable into soup for 5-8 mins. Then
the soup is ready to enjoy.

*Black beans, kidney beans, pinto beans, black-eye peas,
aduki beans, lima beans.*

☞ Soak the beans overnight for less cooking time and less
gas accumulation.
Cook beans for 45 minutes to 1 hour.
Cook in a cast iron or stainless steel pot.

To eliminate gas from beans, prepare beans with ½
cup of ginger juice, or when beans are ready, put a
handful of ginger bark cut up and add to soup while
cooking or use 3-4 pieces of bay leaf.
All beans can also be sprouted for raw food eater.
Check your public library or health food store for an
easy to follow booklet on sprouting.

Sprout Salad

3 cups alfalfa sprouts
3 cups mung bean sprouts
½ cup chopped scallions
½-1 cup red peppers sliced into strips

Combine the above with one of the following dressings:
☞ Mix equal parts of olive or sesame oil and organic apple cider vinegar. Add tamari sauce or Dr. Bronner's Soya Sauce to taste.
☞ You may also use an oil and vinegar dressing (without sugar or additives) from your local food coop.

Marinated Vegetables with Tofu Chunks

1 cup of sliced or diced red onions
1 cup of sliced white onions
1 cup snow peas
1 cup broccoli
Diced tofu
2-3 tablespoons tamari sauce, or to taste
Sage or other herbs that you enjoy.

☞ Marinate the ingredients for a few hours or overnight. Serve on a bed of green leaves and garnish with red or yellow peppers.

Avocado Dip

2 avocados
2 cups of unsweetened tomato sauce
or 2 chopped tomatoes
2 tablespoons miso (fermented soybeans)
2 cups water

☞ Blend and place in a serving dish. Place celery and carrot sticks around the tray to use as a dipper. For heavier eaters, use blue corn chips or seaweed chips.

Winter Fruit Salad

3 yellow pears (diced)
3 apples (diced, but remove skins if waxed)
1 cup walnuts (soak for a few hours or overnight for greater digestion)
1 teaspoon cinnamon powder
4 tablespoons wheat germ (sprinkled over salad)

Five Minute Laxative Soup

*3 cups okra**
1 cup parsley (high in iron)
½ cup leeks and / or onions (good for high blood pressure)
1-2 cups vegetable bouillon
1 teaspoon cascara sagrada

* Acts as both laxative and rejuvenator for genitals.

☞ Add the above ingredients for 3-4 cups of water. This soup takes 5 minutes to prepare.

Uncooked Desserts

Uncooked Pie Crust

2½ cups ground sesame seeds
2 tablespoons sesame oil
1 teaspoon raw maple syrup
1 tablespoon warm water
1 teaspoon natural vanilla extract

☞ Mix with hands and press into sesame-oiled pie pan.

Pie Filling 1

2 chopped pears (remove skin)
2 chopped apples (remove skin)
½-1 teaspoon cinnamon

2 tablespoons maple syrup
¼ cup raisins

☞ Let the above ingredients marinate overnight. Spoon
onto pie crust and top it with 2 tbsp. of wheat germ.
Decorate with well ripened sliced bananas and sliced
strawberries.

Pie Filling 2

1½ cups sliced strawberries
1½ cups blueberries
1½ cups raspberries

☞ Combine ¼ cup of each berry with ¼ cup water and 2
tablespoons maple syrup. Blend and pour over the
remaining berries that have been put in the pie crust.
Cover with ½ cup freshly grated coconut and ½ cup
chopped walnuts.

Chapter 10

Afrikan-Caribbean Meals
by Najami Lezama

I am a firm believer that "You are what you eat" and "Your health is your wealth."

Najami Lezama is a massage therapist, fast therapist, exercise instructor, involved in the performing arts for over 10 years. Now working in the field of healing arts, she conducts massage workshops for adults, children and babies.

Three Breakfast Ideas

Day 1 — Wake Up Oats

> *l cup of raw oats*
> *1 quart of water or soy milk*
> *1 or 2 pieces of papaya*
> *2 dates* (optional)
> *2 oz. raisins*
> *¼-½ cup mixed nuts** (optional)
> *Dash of nutmeg*
> *Dash of cinnamon*
> *1 banana†*
> *Few pieces of dried apple or ½ of fresh apple*

† Bananas should have spots on them so that, instead of being in their starchy state which will cause you gas and constipation, they are in their natural sugar state.
* Soak overnight for easier digestion.

☞ Combine all the ingredients. Bring to a boil a quart of water or vanilla or carob soy milk. Pour hot liquid over other ingredients. Mix well and enjoy.

☞   One can mix lecithin and powdered Brewer's yeast for more variety, or one can use other fruits. Experiment and create different tastes.

A quick easy nutritious breakfast will fill you up and give you energy throughout the day.

Day 2 - Fruit Breakfast

1 grapefruit diced
3-4 slices of pineapple
1 orange
½ cup cherries
½ cup grapes

Have a healthy fruit combination to start off your day.

Day 3 — Pick Me Up

1 cup of freshly prepared pineapple juice
1 cup of freshly prepared orange juice
1 tbsp. of Spirulina (you can substitute chlorophyll)
1 teaspoon of Dong Quai (a Chinese herb)

A delicious powerful health drink to start of your day.

Three Lunch/Dinner Ideas

Day 1 — Melange Supreme

1 or 2 eggplants (melange)
1 cup of water
1 or 2 sprigs of thyme
2 cloves of garlic
2 tablespoons of garlic oil

☞ Wash and cut eggplant into cubes. Chop garlic and ginger; saute in oil until brown. Add eggplant, thyme, a cup of water and cook until eggplant is tender and completely mashed. Add seasoning to taste or a pinch of cayenne pepper if one likes it hot. One can serve this over rice with vegetables and a salad.

Note: Always serve a smaller portion for your dinner meal.

Day 2 — Lentil Soup

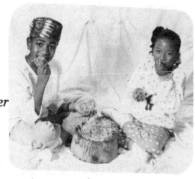

1½ cups of lentils
1-2 potatoes
2 sprigs of thyme
2 cloves of garlic
1 piece of chopped ginger
1 onion
2-3 scallions
1 cup of pumpkin
1 tablespoon of olive oil
Spike seasoning or any veggie seasoning

☞ Wash lentils and put lentils in half a pot of water with garlic, ginger, thyme, oil and seasoning. When lentils are halfway soft, wash potatoes, green bananas and pumpkin. Peel and cut into chunks potatoes, green bananas and pumpkin.

Day 3 - Trinidad Callaloo

16-20 dasheen or eddo leaves (found in most Caribbean vegetable stores)
2 pkgs. of spinach or 2-3 bunches of fresh spinach
½ cup pumpkin
4 tbsps. of olive oil or any unsaturated oils
2 blades of scallions
1 tbsp. butter
8-10 okras
1 large coconut or 2 tbsps. creamed coconut
1 green hot pepper
1 onion
1 sprig of thyme
½ pot of water

☞ Wash leaves and break into small pieces. Cut up okra. Grate coconut, add 2 cups of hot water and extract coconut milk; or use the 2 tablespoons of creamed coconut. Place ingredients in pot (put in the hot pepper whole) and leave to boil until leaves are tender and okra seeds are pink. Use a low fire. Swizzle or use a blender for a quick second. Put mixture back into pot and simmer. Add seasoning to taste.

Note: Do not blend in the hot pepper; the hot pepper is for flavoring. Put it back in when the callaloo is simmering.

This callaloo dish can be enjoyed as a soup by itself or one can incorporate a variety of dishes into the meal, e.g., steamed or boiled corn, brown rice, steamed or boiled plantains (green or yellow) or young green bananas, or a salad.

"MAMA AFUAS"
Children's Food for Holistic Living

Vegetarian foods help prevent childhood illnesses. Simple supper suggestions include:
* Soyaburger on a whole wheat bun and sprouts;
* Soyafrank on whole wheat and sugarless mustard;
* Spinach or whole wheat spaghetti with grated tofu and tomato sauce with soya sauce for taste.

Have a glass of vegetable juice 1 hour before each meal. Eat a large salad with every meal.

Children's Lunches

Monday   Tofu sandwich on sprouted whole wheat bread (tofu cake, 1 tablespoon unsalted mustard, tamari to taste; blend and spread on bread; top with lettuce or sprouts).

Tuesday   Vegetables in a pita pocket. Add lettuce, grated carrots, sprouts, grated beets. (*optional*: tahini butter or avocado spread.)

Wednesday   Raw almond or peanut butter on rice or sesame cakes or whole wheat bread.

Thursday   Vegetable soup in a thermos jug with sea-
            weed crackers.
Friday   Soy burger on whole wheat bun with sugar-
            less and saltless catsup.

In lunch box add soy milk, *un*sweetened fruit juices or freshly pressed juices, 1-2 pieces of fruit, 1 oz. raw nuts (soak overnight for easier digestion). You may also add dried fruits in moderation.

Remember to toast all breads that are used.

If your child catches a cold have him/her eat fruits for one or two days and avoid cooked food. Also give your child an herbal laxative after school, as well as one grapefruit each day s/he is ill.

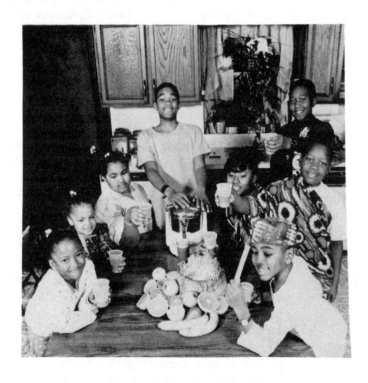

Chapter 11

Nature Cures

A Personal Interview with
Mother Lucille Law (Age 77)
The Mother of Bob Law of Night Talk (WWRL Radio)

Mother Law expressed her personal experience of being raised with natural remedies when she was a young girl.

"In the springtime when we needed cleaning out, we didn't know what we children were doing but, my father would make the boys go up in the pine trees to get pine cones. My father would put all the hearts of those pine cones in a big pot and pour water over them, steam them and make a tea, adding our homemade syrup as sweetener. We had to take this tea for three nights straight and that cleaned us out. As a result of this, we didn't come down with pneumonia even though we were running around barefoot and kicking up in the cold and what not. Nothing happened to us."

"Then my mother would sometimes call to us and say, 'Go out in the field or out in the woods; I need some kind of root.' I can't even think of some of the roots now, but I do remember a couple of the names of the roots. She would send us out to pick the 'little plants' as she would describe them to us and we listened very well. She would explain 'only the leaves are like that,' or 'the flowers are like this.' We would go out into the woods and come back with all kinds of little weeds and herbs. We would pull them up by the roots. She would look at them and pick out what she needed to make "*nip tea*" for the baby. The baby suffered with teething. She would take some of the other things and make some kind of tea for us. That was the way it

71

was. Whatever that was she never told us. She would just say, 'Come and drink this down,' whatever it was. All we knew was that we got better."

"There was a tea that she would make the girls take when their period was a little slow. She would give us pennyroyal tea. I remember when I went to her. I said, 'Mother Bryant, my period is acting up. It looks muddy or something' She said, 'Nothing is wrong with you but you caught cold. Go to the store and buy some pennyroyal.' I went and bought the pennyroyal, made the tea and it cleaned me out. My period came along normally."

"I came down with diphtheria. I was the only child in the family that had ever been laid up sick. Nobody was sick ... and I caught diphtheria from my sister for she had attended a funeral or something where there was the germ. I was so sick with fever. I could see my chin. It was swollen all the way out. My father went out in the yard and got something that he called mullein and brought these big leaves into the house. He put them in a container with cold water. As fast as he put a leaf on my throat it dried up. In fact, it would turn brown because my fever was so high. He stood by my bed and continually put the leaves on my throat to break the fever. And you know what? He broke the fever with that herb."

"At that time, we would talk to the mothers at the Church. They would tell us what to do and we would get along alright. I was at the Church for a long time. I was saved when I was a teenager. There was so much I didn't know that I had to talk to the mothers about."

Q: Were there any men at that time that you knew who had the same wisdom?
A: I think so. You see, my father had the wisdom about that pine tree and there were other things that he would do. They used to give us black draught. I don't know if they gave it to the younger children. There was a time when they put sulphur in shoes. Now, why, I don't know, but all of us had to wear sulphur in our shoes. After awhile, when the shoes got dirty or whatever, they would put more sulphur in our shoes. We had to wear the shoes

with sulphur until they wore out. When we got another pair the same was repeated."

Q: During cleaning time, were there any specific things you had to do?
A: You mean for our bodies? We got that *pine top tea* in the beginning of the spring. The pine top tea cleaned us out in the spring.

* * *

Mother Law's son, Bob Law, remembers his mother's knowledge and use of natural cures.

"My brother and I were cutting wood and my brother split his foot wide open between the big toe. When Mama ran out, the blood was shooting out. The people wore long aprons, you know, (the mothers did) and she ran out and shouted, 'Bring some towels, bring some rags.' She jumped down on the ground on the boy's foot and she cupped it together and said, *'Go get me some spider wed and get some soot out of the chimney.'* They were the only two things she called for and one of us ran to the chimney and the rest of us went to get the spider webs. Mother took the soot and put it right in that wide open cut that was bleeding. She took that spider web and put it right on top of the soot. She closed it altogether. We tore her apron and she bound the foot. She then put it in bags (what we call *croaker bags* or sack bags). She took that croaker sack, bound that boy's foot up, wiped it, and fixed it real well. She put him in a buggy with a horse and sent him to the doctor by himself. I'm not sure at all what the doctor did, but he did give my brother some stitches. He probably cleaned out all the stuff that my mother put in there, but she had stopped the bleeding. That stuff was to stop the bleeding and she stopped it. My brother would have bled to death. My mother saved his life."

* * *

During the days when Mother Law was a child and we as a people healed ourselves with nature cures, there were no doctors available to us. Thus we followed Divine Laws for healing ourselves — the laws that the Creator gave us "To Be Ye Perfect."

We delivered our babies at home with the midwives or the "mothers of the church." Mothers were natural then. They didn't use bottled milk from cows or goats, or formula manufactured in factories. Babies drank milk fresh from their mother's breasts, as nature intended.

When we got fevers, female problems, aches and pain, or whatever the disease was, we used herbs that grew in the fields, mud from the earth, water from the stream and pot liquid from the greens to heal ourselves, to save ourselves. We were medically independent then; we were powerful then, and drug-free. We took care of each others' children and made them respect their elders at all costs. We kept our marriages and families together no matter what. If we are to regain the strength our elders had we must return to the old ways, our traditional ways, and embrace natural healing.

We must love and respect our Afrikan *bush doctors* [herbalists], our midwives, our spiritualists, and our healers. We are truly equipped to heal ourselves. *As it was in the beginning, so shall it be in the end.* I thank Mother Lucille Law for sharing her experiences with us and reminding us of our ability to "Heal Thyself."

P.S. Mother Lucille Law passed soon after this interview. She was attended by seven ministers who conferred on her the title of *Saint*. It was indeed a honor to have been graced by her presence.

• • •

Cleansing is an Afrikan tradition that was carried over to the Caribbean Islands and the southern part of the U.S. In most families, there was a healer who gathered the children, lined them up and gave them a bush tea or herb tea to purge them weekly or monthly. These healers helped to keep the children and adults free of disease.

While living in rural areas closer to nature, we ate pots of greens and drank bush tea. However, since migrating to the cities we have been eating "fast food" and not getting much exercise, if any at all. Because we live less as collective family units more diseases have been able to enter our bodies.

Healing's Natural to the Folks
born in the Hills of Jamaica

It is our cultural right to heal ourselves. Paulette Herron, age 32, was born and raised in Jamaica. She is the wife of a Rastaman and the mother of three children. While I was in Jamaica, I had a brief interview with Sister Paulette. She shared with me knowledge about some of the herbs common to the Caribbean Islands. Many of these herbs are unattainable in health food stores, although they grow wild in the fields of the Caribbean. Below are some of the herbs Sister Paulette shared with me.

- Fever grass - for fevers
- Dandelion - for colds
- Ram goat regular - for colds
- Donkey weed - for colds
- Scorn the Earth - to strengthen a weak body.

For swelling from a wasp sting, mix three of any different kinds of tea leaves and rub on itchy swelling area to relieve discomfort. Any three teas... what a miracle!

- Sour sap leaves - for worms in children.
- Nervous breakdown - boil young Coconut with Strong Back Root and Irish Moss from the sea.

Peline is a young vegetarian, hard working man born and raised in the hills of Jamaica, who freely shared some of the herbal knowledge that he was born into.

- Strong Back Root to eliminate weakness and pain and "for men who are of no use to their women" as quoted.
- Aloe — for a blood wash out.
- Okra — for fast delivery. (The mother of his son delivered her baby in 1½ hours after labor began. She ate fresh okra from Peline father's garden throughout her pregnancy). "The baby just slipped out at the appointed hour."

- Thyme — for easy birth.
- Cerasee — used for cleaning the colon (relieving constipation); for stomach pain and colds.
- Dry Coconut — to clean out your insides.

When in the Caribbean, Haiti, Afrika or Brazil, visit the local "bush" doctor for natural healing direction and further information.

Nature Cures for Common Health Challenges

Clay

In the beginning God gave to every people a cup of clay and from this cup they drank their life.

Proverbs of Digger Indians

Clay is a "body food" that is nutritious. It stimulates, detoxifies and transforms the skin. According to the National Center of Scientific Research, clay contains: oxides, and the chemical elements of silica, titanium, aluminum, iron, calcium, magnesium, sodium and potassium. From page 30 in the *Essene Gospel of Peace*, on clay we have the following:

I tell you truly, your bones will be healed. Be not discouraged, but seek for cure nigh the healer of bones, the angel of earth. For thence were your bones taken and thither will they return. And the knots of your bones will varnish away, and they will be straightened, and all your pains will disappear.

Queen Afua's Rejuvenating Clay

Contents: green clay, red clover, comfrey herbs and purified water and a touch of mint oil.

Suggested uses

▸ *Beauty Facial:* to remove pimples, toxic lines and black heads. Apply clay. Leave on for 30-45 minutes, Apply cucumber slices to eyes to decrease swelling. During this time lie at a 45°. Wash face upward toward eyes with water or take a shower. Dry face, apply gel from aloe vera plant or use an aloe gel product from a health food store. Take 2 tablespoons of gel from aloe plant and combine with warm water and the juice of a lemon or lime. Drink, for beautiful skin comes from within.

▸ *Draws out aches and pains:* Apply clay with gauze overnight.

▸ *Knits Bones:* Apply with a gauze. Leave on overnight for best results. Shower off in the morning. Stay away from all sugar.

▸ *Strengthens scalp and hair:* Massage aloe in scalp after drying wet hair. Apply clay into scalp and hair for at least 2 hours, then wash with Dr. Bronner's peppermint soap or black soap. Then massage *Queen Aloe's Mist* into scalp.

▸ *Relieves Female Disorders:* Use gauze or cotton swab to insert clay into vagina for 5 hours.

▸ *Whitens teeth and removes plaque:* Rejuvenates diseased or bleeding gums. Massage on gums or brush with non-abrasive toothbrush; allow to rest on gums for 1 hour with or without cotton.

▸ *Draws and cleanses body growth:* Apply with gauze for 1 to 3 hours or better overnight.

For full body clay bath, shower with hot and cold water until totally cleaned, then apply clay over entire body. This procedure will remove dead skin, revitalize and refresh your skin and cleanse clogged pores, so your skin can breathe. For best results while using Rejuvenation Clay, eat fresh fruits, vegetables, and drink live juices and herb teas. No sugar, dairy or fried foods. And take enemas or colonics at least 1-3 times a month during use of clay.

Common Health Challenges

Heal Thyself Formulas I, II and III can be applied to all health blockages listed. Meditation, affirmation and prayer should accompany the healing for full recovery.

Addiction to Drugs/Cigarettes

Herbs: Calamus root, alfalfa, dandelion, rosehips.
Juices: Beets, wheatgrass, spirulina.
Other: Clay pack over your liver.

Acquired Immune Deficiency

Herbs: Dandelion, red clove, chaparrell, alfalfa, golden seal (2 teaspoons).
Juices: Beets, green leafy vegetables, scallions.
Baths: 4-8 lbs. epsom salts.
Other: 2 cloves garlic, Vitamin C-2000 mg., Vitamin B-50 mg., 2 tbsp. spirulina or Heal Thyself Nutritional Formula (3 X a day), wheatgrass (4 oz. daily with qt. of water), live food diet.

Anti-Cancer formula

Herbs: Red clover, chaparrell, comfrey.
Juices: Beets, green vegetables, kale, spinach, etc.
Baths: Warm water bath for 20 mins., then take a shower alternating temp. from warm to cool.
Other: Apply clay pack over cancerous area at least 3-7 times a week. During the last 4-9 days of your fast take Sonne #7 & #9 (Bentonite clay ash). This will provide deeper cleansing of the colon by drawing out longtime toxins. Follow directions on Sonne package. Supplement with two enemas a day.

Arthritis — bone builder

Herbs: Comfrey, oatstraw, alfalfa.
Juices: Turnip (for bones), green vegetables
Baths: Warm water bath; soak 30 mins; total massage
Other: Apply clay over aches and pains. Massage peanut oil on painful areas.

Diabetes

Herbs: Blueberry leaves, golden seal, yarrow, marsh-mallow.

Juices: String beans and all other green vegetable juices (½ cup); cucumber juice (½ cup); 1-2 artichokes; ½ bunch watercress; ½ bunch parsley.

Baths: Salt bath using 2-4 lbs. epsom salt; stay in tub

Other: For 20-30 minutes place a clay application over pancreas; 50% of diet should consist of freshly pressed juices; 50-100% of diet should be raw (uncooked) foods; avoid eating, as in all other cases, when the sun goes down, in order to not overwork the body.

High Blood Pressure

Herbs: Vervain, golden seal (should be taken for only 14 days and then off for 14 days so as not to deplete the B vitamins from the body.)

Juices: Leeks, garlic.

Baths: Warm water bath *without salt.* Soak 15 mins.

Other: 2-3 enemas weekly or colon deblocker 3 times a week. Herbal laxatives and enemas will aid digestion.

Indigestion

Herbs: Peppermint

Juices: ½ cup cabbage

Baths: Warm water bath; soak 20 mins.; massage abdomen.

Other: Drink 3 glasses of lemon water before bath; for exercise, try leg raises (15-25), sit ups and deep breathing.

Men's formula

Herbs: Saw palmetto berries.

Juices: Cherry, cranberry.

Baths: 30-45 mins. in 4 lbs. salt bath; steam baths for 1 hr. to 30 minutes.

Baths: 30-45 mins. in 4 lbs. salt bath; steam baths for 1 hr. to 30 minutes.

Other: Clay packs over reproductive organs, cover with gauze overnight.

Nerve blockage

Herbs: Hops, chamomile, mint.

Juices: Celery, cucumber.

Baths: 2-4 lbs. epsom salt in a hot bath every other day for 30 mins.; sleep right after bath.

Nervous breakdown

Herbs: Valerian (boil 15 mins.), wood betony (steep for 2 hours), gota-kola (feeds the brain).

Juices: Celery, cucumber.

Baths: 2-4 lbs. epsom salt in a hot bath every other day for 30 mins.; sleep right after bath.

Overweight

Herbs: Chickweed, fennel.

Juices: Cucumber, parsley.

Baths: 2 lbs. dead sea salt or 4 lbs. epsom salt, 1 cup ginger (freshly pressed, but only if you do not have high blood pressure).

Other: Lecithin (3 times a day), Heal Thyself Formulas I, II, and III; 30 minutes of daily exercise; fire breaths 100 times (4 rounds).

Respiratory problems (asthma/hay fever/colds)

Herbs: Eucalyptus, mullein

Juices: Scallions, red radishes, pineapple,grapefruits, lemons, oranges.

Baths: Add peppermint or eucalyptus or camphor to bath; rub on chest and back; put a few drops of oil on tongue (with 25 deep breaths).

Other: 50-100 deep breaths (2-3 times a day).

Skin eruptions

Herbs: 1 teaspoon golden seal for a cycle of 14 days on and 14 days off.

Juices:	Beets, green vegetables, kale, spinach, etc.
Baths:	Alfalfa or golden seal bath using 1 qt. of tea.
Other:	Clay bath over entire body, dry and wash; apply aloe gel to skin.

Women's formula

Herbs:	Red clover, goldenrod, comfrey, motherwort
Juices:	Cherry, cranberry
Baths:	30-45 minutes in 4 lbs. epsom salt bath; steam bathe for 15-30 minutes
Other:	Clay packs over reproductive organs, cover with gauze overnight.

Nature Cures for Children

Colds and fevers

Herbs:	Peppermint, fennel, powdered golden seal for 7 days (1 teaspoon to 1 cup of warm water).
Juices:	¼ teaspoon horseradish, 1-2 scallions, 1-2 red radishes; use 1 or 2 of these at a time; grapefruit and orange (equal parts).
Baths:	1 lb. salt bath; add eucalyptus and peppermint oil to child's chest, back, and a few drops to bath.
Other:	*Heal Thyself Formulas* I and III; in most cases, 6 drops kyolic (garlic) or 2 cloves garlic; mustard pack on chest overnight; organic apple cider; fast of 50% vegetable and 50% fruit juice for 2-3 days, and 2 pieces of fruit, if hungry.

The above formula is also good for eye infection (apply clay above and below eyes), and ear infection.

For skin eruptions, cover body with clay one inch thick; let dry for ½-1 hour; shower (alternating temperature from hot to cold); cover with aloe gel from plant. (Check Bach flower remedies or other flower essences for emotional imbalances). Talk with your child often; keep communication open.)

Constipation
Check your child a few times a week.
S/he should eliminate 2-4 times daily.

Herbs: Senna, peppermint.
Juices: Freshly pressed pear, apple, grapefruit, prune
Baths: Warm water bath.
Other: Okra, vegetable salads, sprouts; for exercise,
            use rebounder daily 10 mins.

Hyperactivity Learning disabilities
Herbs: Chamomile, gota-kola.
Juices: 1 celery stalk, ½ cucumber, 3-4 carrots.
Baths: Add 4 teaspoons of chamomile and hops to 1 qt.
            water, steep 4 hours; add to tub; 2 lbs. salt
            bath in warm water.
Other: Vitamin B-15 mg. 3 times a day; Formula I (or
            1 tsp. spirulina) and Formula III, 3 times a
            day; eliminate all sugar, natural and unnatu-
            ral, from diet.

Foods for Internal and External Uses

Here are foods that can be taken internally and externally
for health and beauty. Healing can be fun.

• Sliced cucumbers over eyes.

• To reduce swelling, cover eyes and rest for 15 mins.

• Lemons, limes or grapefruits

• Scrub rough blemished areas of elbows, knees, face and feet. Do not use on sensitive skin.

• Avocado facial

• Cleanses & nourishes skin

• Full body scrub:
1 cup each of water & oats with ½ cup cornmeal.

• Mix together and put in bath. Scrub with loofah or scrub over full body and shower.

The Bob Law Mucus Buster
To eliminate chronic mucus congestion

☞ Blend together: 3 tablespoons of organic apple cider vinegar, juice of one freshly pressed grapefruit, juice of one lemon, and 2 drops of pure peppermint oil.

☞ Drink 4 oz. of warm water after consumption. After drinking, do 50-100 fire breaths (rapid breathing). Take for 7-14 days.

Chapter 12

Hints for Natural Living and Fasting

A don't wait to live formula

Most illnesses are the result of shattered dreams, unful-filled goals, empty promises in one or many areas of your life. To change your karma (action & reaction), do things that make you blissful. Don't wait to live, this is all the life you have. You and your freedom and bliss await your heart at this very moment. Live every moment fully, as if it were your first and last.

As you develop this blissful state, the internal war that's going on within your body temple that takes the form of disease begins to diminish, and your eating habits begin to reflect this process. What we eat relates to our state of mind. For example, when you eat and/or desire fried foods, you are usually angry or bitter. When you desire dairy, you are in need of nurturing. When you desire meat, you are feeling aggressive or you are attract-ing aggression to you. When you are consuming a great deal of starch, it is because you are feeling unfulfilled.

On a positive note, when you eat a lot of fruit it brings out a sweet disposition and bright beautiful thoughts. When you eat green vegetables it brings out and reflects inner peace.

Success activities to develop self and support you on your path to purification and your cleansing lifestyle —:

• Join a health food co-op.
• Form a buddy system or support group.
• Become a member of a health spa.
• Visit a Turkish bath.

- Take food preparation classes.
- Write or recite poetry.
- Take a mini-vacation once a month.
- Do pottery.
- Meditate.
- Go to the theater
- Start your own business
- Dance! Sing! Play! Act!
- Develop a natural healing and spiritual library.
- Have clay facials and clay baths with family members and/or friends.
- Take a field trip with your cleansing buddies to holistic and spiritual bookstores, crystal shops, health food stores and holistic health fairs.

Incorporate these activities into your lifestyle and live by the Heal Thyself Purification Method to accomplish your goals and create success in your life.

Daily Affirmations for Higher Living

Depending on your religion, vocalize the name you use for Creator of the Universe.

1) I practice forgiveness so that I too may be forgiven, for it is the will of the Creator.

2) I practice thanksgiving in all my actions, thought and deeds, for it is the will of Allah.

3) I will walk as gently as a deer and glide as smooth as a bird within the temple walls of my divine home, for it is the will of the Most High.

4) My voice will be just above a whisper and only to be raised in states of divine joy and bliss, for it is the will of the Krishna.

5) I will always strive to be patient, loving and giving for it is the will of God.

6) I will serve graciously, joyfully, peacefully those in need, for it is the will of the Neter.

7) As I begin fasting, I will give my food away to one who is most needy, for it is the will of Yahweh.

8) I will stay in constant prayer in all my thoughts, words and deeds, for it is the will of Olodumare.

9) Whatever goodness I expect from others, I will first be that goodness myself, for it is the will of Jehovah.

10) I will fast 24 hours weekly and 3-7 or 21 days monthly so that I might be an example of the Creator's law, for it is the will of Jah.

11) I will harm no living creature. I accept my vegetarianism. I will not use drugs or alcohol for I must keep my body so pure that I may be accepted in thy sight, for it is the will of Yahweh.

12) I will purify all my words, thoughts, actions for it is the will of Great Grandfather and Great Grandmother Spirit.

21 Affirmations for 21-Day Fast

Day 1   I am no longer angry at my disease. I am now able to "bless my disease away" for my disease has no power over me.

Day 2   I look forward to my healing. I look forward to my daily cleansing.

Day 3   I say *YES* to my personal success in gaining physical, mental, spiritual and economic harmony and abundant health.

Day 4   I liberate myself through purification.

Day 5   I accept 100% healing. I am disease free; it is reflected in my life.

Day 6   I shape my destiny with each thought. I think thoughts of success and know in my soul that nothing is blocking me from my good except myself. I have the power to remove all blocks with fasting and prayer.

Day 7   I release my excess weight in thought, word, body and deed.

Day 8   I live a full happy life without fear.

Day 9   Disease is no longer in my life. My cells, blood, bones, nerves, tissues and arteries are filled with pure joy.

Day 10   I am an inspiration for myself and others.

Day 11   I welcome each day with an open mind and an open heart.

Day 12   No one blocks me from my blessings but me. I release all my blockages and free myself.

Day 13   My purification is the key to my long, healthy and vibrant life.

Day 14   Today I am in perfect harmony with myself and the universe.

Day 15   May I continue to be a shining example of health and wealth in body, mind and spirit.

Day 16   Thank you, Creator, for allowing me to wake up to another day of living for I have another opportunity to make it right.

Day 17   I affirm that my reflections bring me love and joy this divine day.

Day 18   Today I am whole and happy. The Creator is active within me and I am active within the Creator.

Day 19   Each atom within my being is being fed with life-giving juices, herbs and high spiritual thoughts, so all is well within me. I give thanks.

Day 20   I am ecstatic about my healing.

Day 21   I accept purification in my life here and now and for
all eternity.

Use the affirmations as spiritual treatments. Read the
affirmation for the day 3 times a day — at sunrise,
midday, and sunset. As you breathe the affirmation in
your soul and repeat it so that the affirmation and you
become one and the same.

Health Diary

Congratulations on the first day of the Heal Thyself Life
Plan! Purchase a notebook or blank page diary. Fill in your
day to day experiences, If at anytime during your cleansing you have wanted to sing, dance, cry, write poetry, or
shout for joy, then put it down in writing. Use these pages
to express who you are, how you are, and what you desire
to become. In other words, fill these pages with your very
being.

Later, the pages will come to reflect your purification
experience as a term of growth; a daily chapter in the book
of yourself, showing your development from embryonic
stages on through to your ever-blossoming rebirth.

Use colored magic markers to express your experience
for the day. You will see a rainbow chart of your cleansing
life. Apply this color system during your fasting or natural
living program.

BLUE   for a peaceful, balanced day.
RED   for increased energy and power.
PURPLE   for spiritual experience and inner harmony.
BLACK   for normal day, business day.
PINK   for love experience of self or another.
GREEN   for healing experience, financial blessing
            received.

Life Goals to Affirm While Cleansing

While on your cleansing and purification path look at
all areas of your life in which you want to see a change.

Fill in this form with all the goals you wish to achieve. Include as many of these areas as you can, along with whatever else you hope to gain from fasting. ASK AND IT SHALL BE GIVEN. SO BE IT. Continue on this cleansing plan until your goals have been reached.

Business/Professional Goals:

_____

_____

_____

_____

Financial Goals:

_____

_____

_____

_____

Relationship Goals:

_____

_____

_____

_____

Health Goals:

_____

_____

_____

_____

Spiritual Development Goals:

_____

_____

_____

_____

Family/Home Life Goals:

_____

_____

_____

_____

Keep record of all the things you have asked for and note the day and time you received your blessings. Purification is High Science.

Weight Loss Goal

Record Your Progress

Cycle I—1st day
Date: _____
Present Weight: _____
Weight Goal: _____

7th day
Date: _____
Present Weight: _____
Weight Goal: _____

Cycle II — 14th day
Date: _____
Present Weight: _____
Weight Goal: _____

21st day
Date: _____
Present Weight: _____
Weight Goal: _____

Cycle III — 28 day
Date: _____
Present Weight: _____
Weight Goal: _____

35th day
Date: _____
Present Weight: _____
Weight Goal: _____

Cycle IV — 42 day
Date: _____
Present Weight: _____
Weight Goal: _____

49th day
Date: _____
Present Weight: _____
Weight Goal: _____

Supporters

As you cleanse you will notice that your supporters become more supportive and your non-supporters become supporters, and then you can place them on the supporters list or either they will leave your life, for you have cleansed that lower part of their reflection out of your life. As you yourself become a loving supporter of yourself, then and only then will all of life support and love you. The wind, the rain, the sun and snow will all embrace you, for you are pure in heart, body and spirit. You will say, "Dear Creator, may we all have good reflections in our lives, because we humbly follow your laws of living."

Below make a list of your supporters and non-supporters and why they either support or oppose what you are doing. Next to their name write the color they make you feel like when you think of them. See how that color in them changes as you move deeper into your cleansing.

SUPPORTERS   NON-SUPPORTERS

Name: _____   Name: _____
Why: _____   Why: _____
Color: _____   Color: _____
Remarks: _____   Remarks: _____
          _____   _____

Name: _____   Name: _____
Why: _____   Why: _____
Color: _____   Color: _____
Remarks: _____   Remarks: _____
          _____   _____

Name: _____   Name: _____
Why: _____   Why: _____
Color: _____   Color: _____
Remarks: _____   Remarks: _____
          _____   _____

Overseas Travel Health Kit
Don't leave home without it!

• Quart-sized enema bags or herbal laxatives for cleansing once or twice a week. Keeping your body light will add ease and enjoyment to your trip.

- Powdered Spirulina. Take 1-2 tablespoons two times a day to strengthen your immune system and protect against weakness and disease.
- Carry a few lemons until you are able to purchase some in the local market.
- A small citrus juice extractor (saucer-sized, manually operated) in order to squeeze fresh orange, grapefruit, lemon and lime juices.
- Golden Seal powder. 1 teaspoon in warm water two times a week to protect against infections and keep the blood pure.
- Carry spiritual reading materials.

Tropical Traveling "DOs" and "DON'Ts"

Don't Eat:
- Fried Foods — they clog arteries which lead to poor circulation and poisoned blood which results also in red eyes.
- White sugar or cooked honey — they cause poor memory and nervous tension. Sugar eats up the nervous system as well as the bones which results in tooth decay and arthritis. Use raw honey whenever possible, instead of white sugar.

Do Eat:
- Breakfast

Breakfast Alternate
   Juice of 1 lemon, cayenne and 1 cup of warm water.
   Freshly squeezed orange juice using 3-4 oranges.
   Freshly squeezed grapefruit juice using 2 grapefruits.
   Fresh fruit, i.e. papaya or watermelon.
   Oatmeal cereal, 3 times a week. Use raw honey, let it soak in hot water 3 minutes. Don't cook to avoid constipation.

Lunch and/or Dinner
   Coconut water and its meat.
   Twenty mins. later eat, any leaves (vegetables) and okra

soup (use fish, okra, peppers, tomatoes, onions).
Boiled bananas, not fried.
If fish is used for protein, limit to 1-2 times a week and
boil or steam instead of frying.
If you must have starches, take them with lunch or
before 7:00 p.m.
Yams, Fufu 1-3 times a week.
Rice 1-2 times a week; soak rice before cooking or even
better, overnight.
Bread may be taken every other day unless you have
constipation, then avoid bread and starches.
Peanut soup or raw peanuts (ground nuts) soak minutes
before eating.

Do Remember:

We should have at least 2-3 bowel movements a day for
excellent health. If you have only one movement a day
or few times a week then eliminate all starches for 14
days. Remember we carry 5-20 lbs of old impacted waste
that has accumulated in the colon over the years.

Salt baths

Take full body or foot baths at least once a week. Stay
in tub for 20 minutes while massaging body from feet
to head.

Ocean baths

While in Africa and the Caribbean, ocean and salt baths
are a special gift and should be taken as frequently as
possible.

Sand baths

Dig a hole big enough to bury yourself in; cover yourself
with the sand. Bathe inside the "Earth Mother" for
30-60 minutes while recharging from the sun. Exit from
sand and rinse in the ocean. This bath is excellent for
cleansing the poisons from the system, beautifying the
skin and drawing you closer to God.

Chapter 13

Colon Therapy

Colon therapy — also called colon hygiene, colonic or colon leverage — is a thorough form of hydrotherapy (water cure) for the large intestines. It has the ability to restore the entire body system by gently washing the colon clear. Colonic therapy should be administered by a trained colonic therapist. This is someone who knows the proper amounts and temperatures of water to use and appropriate herbal implants and solutions to add to the water for respiration of friendly bacteria in the colon and rejuvenation of tissues. A colonic therapist also knows other essentials of the procedure, such as administering reflexology on the feet, massaging the abdomen and recommending the proper breathing patterns to the person receiving the colonic.

Basically, 10-15 gallons of purified water is used. As when taking an enema, a tube is inserted into the anus. By using more water suspended at a greater height than an enema, the colonic irrigation becomes a deeper and more thorough cleansing. The water flows into the anus, up into the descending colon area, across the transverse colon area, down into the ascending colon area and finally to the cecum. The cecum (the end of the large intestines) is where large amounts of unfriendly bacteria hibernate and can cause harm to the entire body system. There are nerve endings in the colon (large intestines) that correspond to every organ in the body. Therefore, washing the colon provides cleansing and rejuvenation for the other organs as well.

The Colon

During one colonic session 1-5 pounds of old, impacted waste is eliminated. By cleansing the colon, you purge 90% of disease causing-bacteria out of the body. A colonic also cleanses tissues that have been penetrated by poisons. It improves lymphatic circulation.

I especially recommend taking a colonic or a series of colonics during the time of seasonal changes to keep the body functioning at top performance. Depending on your needs and state of health, the use of colonic therapy, along with my other recommendations for purification and natural living, should put you on your path to Healing Thyself.

There are connective points in the colon which correspond with the various inner organs of the body. As you cleanse the colon with the use of colonic irrigation (hydrotherapy), you begin to heal those various diseased areas of the body. Colonic irrigation along with nutritional guidance and healing exercise can eliminate diseases such as:

high blood pressure   edema
skin eruption   asthma
headaches   hay fever
Fe/male genital disorders depression.

Tumors and cysts located in the female reproductive organs and breast are in epidemic proportion. In chronic cases, the end result of this health imbalance is a hysterectomy (a complete removal of the uterus) and mastectomy (removal of the breast). With a holistic program of colon cleansing and nutritional guidance, this problem can be eradicated.

Normal bowel movements should be twice a day if you have two (2) small or large meals daily or three (3) eliminations if taking three (3) meals. The body goes through digestive assimilation and elimination with each meal. If this process for any reason does not occur then you have constipation, which means disease is manifesting or has manifested within your physical, emotional and spiritual body. Take plenty of okra if constipated, as well as olive oil with lemon water to alleviate the problem.

Did you know? Jesus (Yoshua) used the gourd and the reed upon a branch of a tree to cleanse his inner parts (colon). Cleanliness is next to Godliness.

Bowel Elimination

The Squatting Posture

The squatting posture is a natural part of the cultures of Afrika, India and China. The squat is applied during times of rest, washing clothes, preparing meals and most of all, for the elimination of waste. In cultures where the squat is used frequently, people generally do not suffer from genital disorders. In western countries such as Europe and America, use of the squat as a relaxant and/or healer is virtually unknown. The result is that people here are suffering a great deal with many of the diseases listed earlier.

As per experience, Queen Afua recommends the use of the squatting stool during elimination. This stool aids the body by elevating the feet when placed in front of the toilet.

The commercial toilets now in use are of hindrance to the natural functions, for the legs are hanging in line or slightly lower than the hips, causing blockage and making the body work harder through straining, resulting in constipation and hemorrhoids.

Use of the squatting technique, as well as the squatting stool is of great importance to aid elimination in the hydrotherapy (bath) room. Better elimination is beneficial toward relief from the above-mentioned ailments.

The Artful Way of Elimination

Step 1:   While sitting on toilet, squat with one or both legs.

Step 2:   Inhale breath for four (4) counts; exhale for

eight (8) counts.

Step 3:   On your elimination while inhaling, fill your being with all the goodness there is.

Step 4:   On the exhale, let go and let God, as you release deeply all the negativity in your body, mind, and spirit.

Then sit very still for a moment and feel the peace of your release.

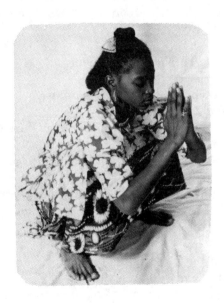

Chapter 14

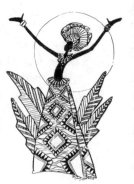

In Celebration of Women:
Full Women Free

All we want to do here is to be full women.
We can't be Full and Free if we drip, drop, drip, drop uhh,
We just want to be as free and full as the Roaring Ocean
The Blazin' Sun & Full Moon and Wide Earth and High
Mountains and Space.

We just want to be Natural Women.

Those women who created the pyramids,
that still stand to the heavens.
Those women who lived off of herbs & bushes &
berries & You, Creator!
Those women who did not bleed. Not the first women.

We want to be free to dance the dances of joy and
sing songs of bliss and say words of power and touch lives
so deep, so sweet.

We don't want no more pain,
We don't want to give no more pain.
No more bleeding, cryin', weepin', moaning.
I can't use no PMS, no more tumors resting in my nest!

I'm gonna free me from my bondage and
who said I gotta be cursed anyway?

Oh, it's that cycle again.

Oh goodness, oh gracious.
There's a war going on in me!
Uhh, I've been wounded 1, 3, 5, 7 days!

Oh no don't take my womb!
Give me back my womb! My nest!
I gotta swirl with my nest. A growth!

Leave my breast alone.
Let me be, let me be.
I gotta dance with my breast.
All I want to do here and now is to be
Full Women Free.

Natural Women, Women Sacred, Women Divine,
Women Loving, Women Gracious, Potent and Kind,
Women Clean, Women Whole, WOMEN HEALED!

Whatever you want to be as a Woman, go on and be.
Can't nobody put no limits on me!

If you want to be an Artist, go on and be.
If you want to be a Scientist, go on and be.
If you want to be a Mother who's a Writer, go on and be.
If you want to make soup, or own a business or
do cartwheels down the street, go on and be.

Being you're so powerful, so purified, so spiritual.
You can be anything you want to be!
If you want to be President of a country,
child, go on and be.

Whatever I wanna do & be ...
Mother, Father, God already gave it to me.

We women just want to be and we're going to be and
We are Full Women Free.

Cause if I don't feel full within myself,
l just might lose myself;

and I love you Free Women.

I don't want to lose any of you.
l love all of Me!
Free Women, go on and be!

FREE

Be Healed.

This poem is dedicated to Heal Thyself Women's Research Group for Living a Pure Life.

For their efforts of constant purifying for a period of one to seven months on fruits, vegetables, live juices, and monthly fasting, prayer and constant purification of the soul, thoughts and heart.

For believing, knowing and living the truth that women need not bleed and suffer monthly and had the power to bring their menses from 6 days to 4, from 4 days to 1.

Thank you for being a living witness and enduring until the end:

Kamari Aduke	Pearl L. Boissiere
Merlene Byron	Arlene Crosby
Jacquelyn Crossland	Khadijah Dunn
Shirley Edwards	Etherine Fortune
Lynda Johnson Garrett	Colleen Goldberg
Deanna Hope	Tracy Jerigen
Isa Karriem	Marcia Lilly
Akua Morris	lbon M. Muhammad
Omani Peterson	Khadijah Rahman
Joy Jon San (*Illustrator*)	Fikriyyah Sharrief
Mimi Strum	Shaunderion White
Adamen (Lenora Peterson)	

And for Elder Micah for inspiring this sacred cleansing program so that other women would no longer have to suffer.

Special thanks to the Mothers of Purification: Queen

Esther, Lady Prema, Dr. Abena Asantawaa, Mother Lucille Shephard, and Fatimahta Adegoke.

Choices

These words will be found in the screenplay, *In All My Born* by Ayoka Chenzra. A mystic healer (played by Queen Afua) speaks these divine words to a young female child just coming into her woman-ness and letting her know she has choices to be well and whole or ill, imbalanced and in pain.

"You are a woman. This is a most sacred time for you; a time of renewal, a time for power. Women of old did not suffer. They would go to themselves, and pray, heal, receive spiritual messages for guidance and give thanks for their woman-ness."

"The modern woman with her impure lifestyle suffers during her moon 4, 5, 6, 7, and sometimes 8 days."

"During your monthly moon, a message from the pituitary goes down to the ovaries and tells them to release an egg which travels down the fallopian tubes. If your body is free from toxins, then you release a white milky fluid; but if your body is full of poisons from devitalized processed foods and bad thoughts, then you may suffer for days and days."

"Rainbow," the mystic said to the young woman, "you must lead a clean, healthy life, or else when you reach my age you will suffer with tumors, cysts and early aging."

"I love you, Rainbow. Take care."

Queen Afua

WHERE ARE YOU?
Are You A Full Woman Free?

Over the years I've found a direct relationship between dietary habits and the health of female organs.

Note that as we travel down the recommendations, it indicates a breakdown of women's health and a decline of healthy living.

Ideal Health

☞No female problems (vaginal disorders)
Menses for 1-3 days
Inner peace and harmony

- Whole Foods, fasting, enemas, herbs
- Daily exercise
- No flesh or fried foods
- Limited starches
- Bowel movements 3 or more times a day; stools long, light-colored, full and easy to eliminate

Decline of Health

Beginning Stages of Degeneration

☞Prolapsed colon causes prolapsed uterus which induce lower back pain which results in 3-5 day menses which causes vaginal itch/discharge.

- Flesh foods (fish, chicken), night-time eating, lack of exercise
- Diary and starches
- Two or fewer bowel movements

2nd Stage of Degeneration

☞Cysts and fibroid tumors
Caesarean section (difficult birthing)
Lack of sexual orgasm (due to blockage/poor circulation)
Menses of 5-8 days or acute menses of 8 days to 2 weeks

- Flesh foods (beef, pork).
- Drugs (orthodox and unorthodox)
- Continued neglect of exercise
- Dairy, starch, sugar
- One bowel movement: short, hard stool
- Kidney stones

3rd Stage of Degeneration

☞Tumors (hysterectomy)
Removal of the uterus; sterility
Lack of sexual enjoyment or stimulation
Suppressed emotions; discomfort with femaleness

*   Continued negligence of emotional physical condition
*   One bowel movement a day or a few times a week, hard short grassy

Vaginal Regeneration

Women, stop feeding your tumors. Save your uterus and save your breasts.

Foods that create and feed tumors or cysts are flesh products such as all meats (pork, beef, chicken and fish), dairy products such as milk, cheese and ice cream). Avoid fried foods and starches.

A diet heavy in these foods creates 4-8 days or up to 2 weeks of bleeding. Usually, when a woman receives surgery to remove a tumor or cyst, it grows back in 1-2 years because she, in her ignorance, continues to eat the above-mentioned foods.

Once she eliminates the above foods, the tumor either will be eliminated or will not develop again. If a woman has a tumor or cyst and she discontinues eating foods that help a tumor or cyst to strive, the tumor or cyst begins to die out and comes out of the woman through the vagina in small or large lumps of what appears to be mucus.

The regeneration and purification process is speeded up if she takes large amounts of vegetable juices, spirulina, wheatgrass and women's herbal formula of goldenrod, comfrey, red clover, red raspberries, don quai (a Chinese herb that strengthens the uterus, builds blood and is high in Vitamin B_{12}).

Add 3 teaspoons of each herb to 3-5 cups of water. Steep over night. Strain and drink in the morning.

Basic Regeneration Diet consists of:
- Live fruits and vegetables, vegetable broth and vegetable soups.
- Please, no starch, even if whole grains, until problem is totally eliminated.

Bless Your Disease Away

Emotionally, you must consistently release anger, frustration and disappointment out of your vagina and mind. Release thoughts of anyone who you feel has hurt you and take the experience as a lesson. Forgive that person in order for you to release the person or experience out of your womb along with the tumor.

A good time or way to release emotionally and revitalize yourself spiritually is during your healing bath. While in bath, massage, breathe, nurture and bless your pain and disease away. Fill your womb with peace and mentally bathe your womb with green light for healing and pink light for love. Each month thereafter, you will bleed 1 day less. The more you love your vagina and your womaness, the sweeter and more harmonious the children that come through your sacred canal will be. The planet's salvation depends on you loving yourself. It may take you months or years to bring your bleeding from 5 days to 1 day, a half day to 1 hour. But don't give up, for healing is close at hand.

Chant daily and pray for women who have buried their wombs. Women, Heal Ourselves! Save Our Uterus! Save Our Wombs! Save Our Uterus! Save Our Wombs! Save Our Uterus!

In order to receive the Creator's blessing in the heights, we women must be willing to live without flesh and the by-products of the beast. When an animal sheds its blood for our desires, we too shall shed our blood, in this case, monthly for the women. As Kahlil Gibran states in his book, *The Prophet*, "When you kill a beast, say to him in your heart, by the same power that slays you, I too am slain: and I too shall be consumed. For the law that delivered you into my hand, shall deliver me into a mightier hand."

Low Menus / toxic-filled women	*High Menus / purified women*
(Heavy Bleeding)	(Light Bleeding)
3-8 days or more	1-60 minutes to 1-2 days
clotting	no clotting
Depression	Gaiety
Mood Swings	Mental peace, harmony
Loss of vital life fluids	Retention of vital fluids
Low energy	High energy
Agitated	Strong concentration
Infertility	Increased fertility
Poisoned vagina-clotting, odor	Pure odor-free vagina
Quick to anger, violent temper	Healthy happy and beautiful disposition

Depending on the length of your menses, it will deter-mine the intensity of either expression.

If you find that you have cleansed yourself with nature's tools for weeks and months and your tumor is still strong within, and if you choose surgery, your healing after surgery will be expedient. If you live naturally thereafter, your tumor in most cases will not return. Continue in this way for 1-2 years and you will no longer be feeding the tumors and cysts.

Loosen your thoughts, your hips and temple gate. As we enter into our healing and changing our diets, we should also apply this simple message. We must stop constricting ourselves. Take off those tight pants and girdles for improved circulation of oxygen, blood flow and nutritional acceptance. When in the privacy of your home, spread your thighs and allow (Shu) the angel of air to wash your sacred chamber, as you breathe deeply 50 or more fire breaths. During this time, send messages of beauty and love to and through your divine canal. When able, let (RA)the angel of fire (sun) recharge and bathe you with its rays of light and healing. Be at peace with your womanness and observe your healing taking place.

No more hysterectomies. No more drugs. No more surgery. No more pain. I address supreme healing to women as in time of old when we were healthy, happy and whole.

Know that you are a distinctive beautiful flower and a healing herb with breasts and buttocks and a womb. You come with sacred earth medicine to heal yourself. Be not afraid.

A Special Message to Breast-feeding Mothers

You should strive to breast-feed for 1-3 years (if not for the full time, at least part time). Mothers should follow a natural mucus-less diet so that the baby is tree of colic, constipation, constant crying, cradle cap. Mothers should eat fresh fruits, vegetables (especially okra), vegetable juice of 4-5 carrots, ½ cucumber, ½ turnip, and vegetarian proteins such as peas, beans, sprouts, tofu, seeds and nuts. If you are a meat eater, eat only baked non-shell fish.

Take advantage of the following nutrients: TwinLab Yeast Liquid (2 tablespoons), Spirulina (2 tsps. to 2 tbsps.) and 500-1000 mg. of Vitamin C, all to be taken 2-3 times a day. Also utilize vegetarian calcium sources in the form of soya milk, nut and sesame seed milk, carrot and turnip juice, and oatstraw, dandelion, alfalfa, and comfrey herbal teas.

Mothers: Take steam baths to keep the pores cleansed and the nerves relaxed. If mother is upset, she will poison the baby. So, husbands, nurture and love the mother of your child, the love of your life.

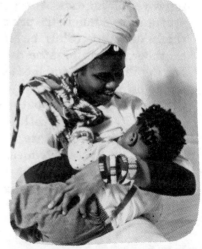

Here are some other things the brothers can do:

- Prepare her bath once a week and place her into the tub. Remember: to serve is to be served.
- Bring her flowers.
- Massage her gently with 3 parts olive oil, 1 part Vitamin E.

Tahema's Formulas
for Pregnant Women

1) 3 parts red raspberry, 2 parts nettle, 1 part anise — to make childbirth easier. This is high in iron, calcium, and other minerals.
2) For easier labor, utilize this formula for 4-6 weeks before delivery and during labor: red raspberry, squaw vine, black cohosh tincture and anise for sweetener.

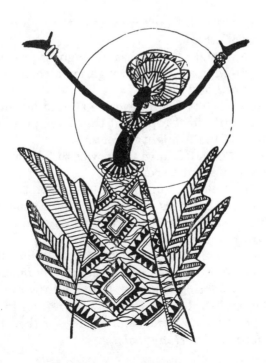

The 12 Principles of Divine Sacred Woman

These 12 Principles are for women who strive to be
healed and whole. The woman is the center of the home.
If she takes on her sacredness of womanhood, the children
and husband (mate) will also be functioning in Divine
Order.

As you affirm these principles daily for yourself, you will
steadily experience yourself opening up like that of a
beautiful lotus.

AS A SACRED WOMAN: I am the highest physical and
spiritual projection of *woman-consciousness*. I represent the abundance of life in health, wealth, love and
beauty.

AS A SACRED WOMAN: I embody grace, dignity and
majesty at all times.

AS A SACRED WOMAN: I epitomize the highest aspects of
the feminine principle in my great love of being a
Woman.

AS A SACRED WOMAN: I nurture myself through the
nurturing of others.

AS A SACRED WOMAN: I manifest the highest principles
of *spirit, mind*, and *body*, through my alchemy of
thought, word and *deed.*

AS A SACRED WOMEN: I can never be abused by *man,
woman* or *child* for I represent the active presence
and power of the Almighty Creator.

AS A SACRED WOMAN: I have the power to *heal* with a
glance, a *smile* or a *word.*

AS A SACRED WOMAN: I am the ORIGINAL HEALER, who
calls upon my brothers and sisters, (the Elements
AIR, FIRE, WATER AND EARTH) to heal *physically,
mentally and spiritually,* for I am the
Great-Granddaughter of MOTHER NATURE herself!

AS A SACRED WOMAN: I beam and radiate my *inner*
Divinity, by adoring my *outer* Being with garments
befitting my Royal form. I would never dress in the
clothing of my masculine counterpart, for then I
surrender my power! my tools!

AS A SACRED WOMEN: I don't kill living creatures for food. I am a vegetarian-fruitarian by nature, my food contains the breath of life. I take into my body temple live fruits, vegetables, nuts, seeds, juices and herbs for "life comes only from life; life gives only unto itself."

AS A SACRED WOMAN: I endeavor to transform my domestic atmosphere into a PARADISE!!! My environment radiates my inner tranquility. The very walls of my home (temple) engender the divine sanctity and safety of the womb. So whoever enters into the temple shall be lifted to their heights.

AS A SACRED WOMAN: I am ever striving to resurrect and exalt the divinity of my mate and counterpart. I recognize that my inner balance must manifest externally in my relationship with MAN, if the true potential of the Higher Self is to be made known to me.

Upon each rising and setting of the sun I affirm these 12 Principles so that I may be living more each day, the heights and the perfection of the Divine Sacred Woman.

I, _____, accept my divine position and responsibility as a Divine Sacred Woman on _____.

"Shine You Brilliant Woman, First Mother, Healer, Lover of the Universe."

Chapter 15

Hydrotherapy: Water Baptism

Water Purification: An Ancient Ritual

The water element was very sacred with the first civilization of the Nile Valley. The Khamites used a great deal of water for Spiritual Baptisms to wash away the ills, to bring forth life and to prepare one to enter the Mystery Systems, which was the entrance into knowledge of the Most High. To support this, it is said in *Ancient Egypt Light of the World* by Gerald Massey, that we might call the Khamites very particular Baptists. In the first 10 gates into the great dwelling of Ausar — the Resurrection Principle — the initiate is purified at least 10 times over, in 10 separate baptisms, in 10 different waters in which the Neteru had been washed to make the water holy. The initiate would say, "May I be protected by seventy purifications." In the rituals, it is said, "I purify myself at the great stream of the galaxy. That which is wrong in me is pardoned and the spots upon my body, upon the earth are washed away. Low, I come, that I may purify this soul of mine in The Most High Degree." Water is as sacred now, in the Motherland of Afrika, as it was then. When you enter into someone's home, to this day, the first thing you are given is water. Water represents life (Ankh). The oldest word for Life in an Afrikan language is *(NK)* commonly spelled *Ankh*. Nk, is rendered (a wave of water) and (a sieve). This establishes water as a primary element of the Life Force. The sieve catches all impurities.

Researched by HRU ANKH RA SEMAHJ SE PTAH
Sen-ur: HETEP PTAH TEMPLE

Healing Water Prayer

Oh Father, Mother God, these waters that I bathe and
  wash myself in are Spiritual and Holy,
    for they are your Waters.
Baptize me in your Holy Divine Waters.
  Direct my course as I cleanse with this Purifying Tool.
Purify me, Oh Creator of the Universe.
  Cleanse me from within and without.
Help me to let go of all that is not you;
  all that is not truth.
Allow this Holy Water to scrub all my sickness, pain and
  confusion away.
I now wash my head and there is light.
  I wash my heart and there is love.
I wash my body temple, so that I may be drawn closer and
  closer to you.
Hold me in your arms, Great & Divine Father, Mother.
  Baptize me with your Love.
Heal me with your Love.
  Engulf me with your water.

Queen Afua

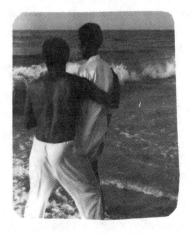

Apply this prayer with the fire (sun) bath, earth (clay or sand) bath, air bath and water (ocean) bath.

This Water Prayer is dedicated to Baba Ishangi for teaching me the ancient Afrikan Power of Spiritual Bathing. Pray before and during your water healing (baths, enemas, colonics, nose rinses and showers). In place of Father, Mother God, put in the term you use for The Most High.

A Few More Words About Water...

I recommend that you read *Colon Health* by N.W. Walker. Mr. Walker, as myself, was a colon therapy student of Dr. Robert A. Wood, a healer who lived to the age of 88 and was going strong to the end.

My study under Dr. Wood, as well as my personal health experience, have led me to understand and be very grateful for the element water. I suggest and constantly use many forms of water therapy. Colonics, baths, showers, nose rinses, enemas, eye washes, sponge baths, drinking large amounts of water, sitz baths, foot soaks, steam baths, indigenous American sweat lodges, showers in waterfalls, all are ways of cleansing oneself, inside and outside.

Very late one night while she was editing this section, Gerianne shared with me some thoughts she had about water: "They are all connected, the waters. Whatever water cures are used, on whatever parts of the body, they are all connected. Like the old 'knee bone connected to the shin bone' thing we used to sing as children. Every 'water thing' we do can be 'hydro-therapeutic.' And that only makes sense because aren't all the waters of the earth also connected? The snow on the mountaintop becomes a stream, a waterfall and then after a while, a river and after that an ocean and fog and rain and then snow again. Around and around we go and are healed. Isn't God wonderful?"

Baths

Soaking in a warm tub will enable the body to release toxins through the skin. Epsom salt or dead sea salt is recommended (unless you have high blood pressure). Use 2-4 lbs of salt and soak in tub for 30 minutes. A few drops of eucalyptus oil is recommended for general use and especially when there is congestion in the lungs. If you have a cold or mucus congestion, massage peppermint or camphor oil into your chest while bathing. Also, add a few drops into the bath water. See the following chart and refer to *Chapter 3* for suggested oils in bath.

Scrub body with loofah brush and wash with natural soap or Queen Afua's Rejuvenating Clay to open and cleanse pores and allow the body to breathe. You can massage your feet and body during your bath, always working upward toward the heart.

Take warm bath daily. Follow with brisk cool shower. (Eliminate cool shower if you have a cold or respiratory problems. Substitute with a warm shower.) Dry body well and anoint with oil.

To set the stage for profound self-healing, do the following: Place a small candle to light the way in the hydrotherapy (bath) room. Also place fresh flowers to beautify your transcendental experience. Burn frankincense and myrrh or sage brush for spiritual cleansing.

Bath oils to consider:

Almond oil - for prosperity.
Camphor - to strengthen psychic/spiritual powers.
Honeysuckle - to promote quick thinking and aid memory.
Hyssop - to purify the atmosphere and the body; increases
    finances.
Rose oil - for love matters; to inspire peace and harmony.
Spikenard - wear during rituals to the ancient deities of
    Egypt (Khamit); also anoint sacred objects, such as
    altars, tools, etc.

How to take an Enema

It is of utmost importance to take a daily enema while on this cleansing. A quart-size enema bag will be sufficient. Fill the bag with warm water. Be sure to test the water temperature on the inside of your wrist. You may want to add 3 tablespoons of organic apple cider vinegar to combat symptoms of respiratory disorders.

Other enema implant suggestions include:

☞ Wheatgrass Enema: Add 1 oz. to 1 quart of water.
Liquid Chlorophyll: Add 3 tbsp. to 1 qt. water.
Lemon/lime Enema: Add juice of 1 lemon/lime to 1 qt. of water. First remove seeds.
Garlic Enema: Empty 2 capsules of garlic or 6-12 drops of liquid Kyolic into 2 qts. of warm water, then into enema bag and mix well.

☞ Lubricate the nozzle tip of a 1 or 2 quart enema bag with K-Y Jelly or the like.

☞ Lie in the tub on your back or on your left side. Insert nozzle into rectum and take in ½ to 1 cup of water.

☞ Massage the lower left side of your abdomen. Work especially hard on any lumps or rigged area that you might feel — these are deposits of fetal matter.

☞ After 3-4 minutes of massaging let in more water. Continue to massage across the abdomen and down the right side. This is where the greatest problems occur, so be especially thorough in massaging this area.

☞ Do not retain the liquid if you feel the need to eliminate. Move to the toilet and release. Then repeat the procedure.

☞ While sitting on toilet to eliminate, massage abdominal area from right to left, breathe deeply while inhaling and exhaling.

Most people will expel brown or gray mucus, black fleck-like matter, parasites, and other surprising matter.

For deeper cleansing of old impacted waste, place a stool in front of toilet, place both feet flatly on stool or sit directly on the toilet seat in the ancient position of a squat.

We must work on our colon through cleansing, enemas, abdominal exercise, proper breathing and prayer until we have 3 bowel movements daily. Once our colons are cleansed, 90% of all disease will no longer plague our bodies.

My cleansing proverb: *Life is a reflection; if you don't like your life, wash your mirror.*

Nose Rinse

If the nasal and sinus passages are unclear, it hinders the flow of oxygen to the brain. This lack of oxygen also affects the eyes and ears. So, clear your nasal and sinus passages and enjoy clearer vision, greater hearing, and a sharper mind.

To prevent and relieve nasal congestion, do nose rinses frequently.

- Fill a small tea pot or neti pot with ½ to 1 cup of water with a pinch of sea salt, or 1 teaspoon of chlorophyll.
- Tilt your head over the sink so the left side of your face is parallel to the sink. Open your mouth and keep it open.
- Place the nozzle of the neti pot at your right nostril and gently pour the water.

If done correctly, the water will flow through and expel through your left nostril. Repeat this procedure, beginning with the head tilting to the right and pouring water into the left nostril, expelling through the right.

Following the nose rinse, do 25-50 full fire breaths.

Chapter 16

Bodywork: Exercise, Massage and Yoga

**Daily exercise is necessary for a
minimum of 15 minutes to a maximum of 1 hour.**

Basic Head-to-Toe Exercises

Full Body Breath — deep inhalation on a count of 4. Exhale on a count of 8. On the inhalation, extend the abdomen out along with expansion of the chest while relaxing the shoulders and the rest of the body. As you exhale, contract the abdomen and release the chest. With each breath relax the body and the mind deeper and deeper.

☞ As you do any form of exercise, always apply this deep breath to pump life into the blood, nerves, arteries, muscles, lungs and brain. When moving arms, legs or head upwards inhale. When you move any part of the body downwards, exhale.

☞ Visualize your pores of your skin opening and closing with each breath. Do this full body breath; breathing from head to toe at least 25 to 100 or more times.

☞ Fire Breathe — For more energy, and increased circulation for mental power, and physical strength. Inhale and exhale rapidly using the abdomen as a quick release pump. Complete 25-100 breaths.

☞ Legs in 45^0 against the wall (natural slant board) 5-10 minutes. Sit ups and leg raises 10-20 times.

☞ Arm swings 20-40 times front and back in circles and sides.

☞ Daily walking — 15 minutes — swing your arm as you walk for upper body circulation.

116

☞ Neck rolls — 4 times both sides: Shoulder lifts — 10-20 times.

☞ Pelvic lifts — sitting on your back, bend your knees in to prevent lower back pressure. With each movement up you inhale; with each movement down you exhale. *Example:* As your arm moves up towards the ceiling, you inhale the breath; as your arm goes down towards the floor, you exhale.

The breathing process is the same with each movement in all exercise forms.

MASSAGE FOR RENEWAL
by Deanna N. Hope

The origins of therapeutic massage are rooted in the common instinctual response to hold or rub a hurt or pain. Massage as an art is as old an civilization itself. (When I say old I mean Afrika old). It has been used for thousands of years for relaxation and restoring and promoting health. In some countries it is even a medical discipline.

In the last ten years, the United States has begun to recognize massage as one of the most viable means of stress reduction available. (These people are very slow.) Revitalized, tired muscles feel like they have had an extended rest. Often times massage can be used when sleep time is limited.

You will feel after a good massage like you have had a good night's rest. You may even admit to feeling younger. Massage relieves tension, lowers stress levels, improves mental response, increases cardiovascular and internal organ efficiency, flushes out metabolic toxins, and reduces recovery time from injuries.

We are fortunate beings in that we are directly involved in the "goings on" of our own bodies. We are the best doctors for our own aches, pains and cures. The more in tune you become with yourself, the easier it is to divert discomforts, detect the cause, and direct the cures. As a society at large we are not taught to be our own doctors or healers.

A generation has passed in which the treasure of home-grown cures of our legacy of Afrikan knowledge instilled in our genes and our elders, grandparents or greatgrandparents is bypassed for the "quick fix" of the local "drug" store. The more attention we give to this great reserve of intuitive knowledge we will spend less time and money on doctor's bills.

Massage as a healing art-form is one of those great treasures. It can be as simple as getting a hug to spending hours, if needed, giving yourself a massage, as part of your at home healing treatment. The more time spent caring and getting to know every part of your body, mind, and spirit, the less time you'll spend doing things that limit your health, strength, and vitality, and believe me, all around you will help you in maintaining the good practices that you follow and emulate your example.

Sounds to me like the beginning of bright and beautiful new world. Anyone who knows me well can tell you I love to get a good massage. The very first professional massage I received was so magnificent I enrolled in a one-year course to obtain my license and certification.

The best way I can describe the benefits of massage is to tell you the many ways it can help you in overcoming debilitating aches, pains, and stresses. One of the first things to remember when you are getting a massage is the importance of relaxation. Both you and the massage therapist will enjoy the fullness of the benefits of the treatment if you relax your mind, body and spirit.

Massage is a very spiritual as well as a physical and mental healing therapy. Our ancestors of ancient Khamit knew well the benefits of this ancient healing art. They studied the body in all aspects — spirit, mind and body — and understood that the balance of the chakras (energy points) and meridians (highways to connect nerve cells) were key in the developmental and healing processes of the body. They were cognizant that our self-concept, in body, mind and spirit, affected our breathing which affected our life and health.

They also developed many other healing art-forms which were later inherited by other cultures that we know today.

For instance, what is called Hatha Yoga today comes from the ancient Khamitic form called Het-Hru Yoka.

Basically, the form is centered around the breath or technique of breathing, which is life. Once our breath is centered, through the MRKHT (pyramid) of the nose and diaphragm, all the other areas of the body is also centered. The spirit which is our earthly connection to the divine creator and knower of all things is continually in communication with our Ba (spirit) and our Ka (soul) to manifest its divinity in our Kaat (body).

From pre-conception to birth to all of the stages of our growth and development, the spirit divinely guides our Kaat to develop to the highest physical, mental and spiritual potentials. Whether it be in art, science, dance, or any form the Creator manifests, our Ka (soul) must be attuned or at one with the Divine Spirit in order to develop to the unlimited potentials of the Creator.

As the IAU Khrishna-Christos stated, "Greater things will ye do than me." Therefore the art, and science of massage and HET-HRU Yoka breath therapy facilitates the manifestation of the Kaat (body) to the Divine Spirit.

As we begin life even before conception and growth through childhood and puberty to adulthood, our bodies changed as our mental development grew with the ideas and information our parents, families, and institutions of learning supplied.

It may be very apparent to you how differently the body develops of people born in different areas of the globe. Not only because of climate, but also because of diet and spiritual mentality as well. One can sometimes clearly place a Western "civilized" physique to that belonging to one of an Afrikan or other person of closest Afrikan Ancestry. We can attribute this most readily to the spiritual development of the person in relation to the adaptation of the individual to the Divine Spirit.

Given the above, without the proper attention given to healthy nutritional habits such as cleansing, fasting, or drinking water, fruit and vegetable juices, and of divine spiritual development, as opposed to religious barbarism, a person will develop the physika (physical and spiritual bodies) to match whatever stage the above has revealed or manifested.

Poor spiritual development, lack of proper cleansing and fasting or unhealthy nutrition will manifest the same in illness and disease, aches, pains and stress. Therefore, proper intuitive spiritual guidance, cleansing, fasting, and eating, plus massage and exercise, Het-Hru Yoka (breathing) will facilitate the transformation of our divinely given bodies into vehicles of divine light energy and supreme power.

It is the Divine will of the Creator that at 20, 30, 40, 50, 60 70, and so on, we should feel at maximum physical potential and divine strength as we did at 20 years of age or even better. The cells in our bodies regenerate entirely every seven years. We can help our bodies to continue this regeneration process by continuing to exercise our Divine Breath in Het-Hru Yoka. Divine touch is massage and divine thinking is true Maat Tehuti, Spiritual Wisdom. The at-one-ment of our spirit, mind and body with the Maat Hru, True Vision and Wisdom will match our physika as well. "And the corruptible will put on incorruption" all in Divine Time.

Here is a list of some of the known benefits of massage:

- Opens blood vessels to improve circulation.
- Increases blood supply and nutrition to muscles.
- Greater ease and range of motion.
- Stimulates lymphatic system to help filter bacteria.
- Assists in maintaining chiropractic adjustments and alignments.
- Aids in stress reduction.
- Increases longevity.

In addition to the benefits of massage, there is one overall objective to keep in mind at all times — and that is love.

Most definitely, without love for yourself and life, any amount of massage, exercise, fasting, cleansing, or purifying will help to a good degree. These efforts are aided a thousand-fold when we do it with love. The Great

Spirit most definitely helps those who make any effort to help themselves.

Love yourself and know that you are here because of the Love of the Great Spirit who wanted you to be here to enjoy life to its fullest and breathed the breath of life into your soul to make you a living, vibrant and beautiful being.

There are many techniques for massages. In looking for a masseur or masseuse, one should keep in mind the following objective: the importance of a loving, giving, sharing spirit. It is also very important to remember that you get what you put out. We are all reflections of one another.

Here are some massage techniques that you can look for in a therapist or if you are interested in studying a technique on your own.

Swedish Massage

Swedish massage is the systematic and scientific manipulation of the soft tissues of the body. In 1812, P. Henrik Ling, a Swedish physiologist, developed Swedish massage by applying scientifically established principles of anatomy and physiology to Chinese techniques and combining them with the movements of Swedish gymnastics. The Swedish massage therapist uses kneading, stroking friction, tapping, and sometimes shaking and vibrating parts of the body in order to stimulate circulation, increase muscle tone and create a balance within the structure and function of the muscular, nervous and circulatory systems. In Swedish massage the general purpose is to increase circulation, remove toxins and improve flexibility and tone the muscles. The therapist should begin with slow gliding strokes and gradually increase in vigor and movement of the limbs for increase range of motion.

Shiatsu

Shiatsu ("Shi" = finger, "Atsu" = pressure) is an Oriental massage in which particular points of the body are pressed to ease aches, pains, tensions, fatigue and symptoms of disease. Pressure is applied to these vital points with fingers, thumbs and palms to bring relief. (Great therapists like myself will even use their elbows, knees, whatever works, to remove the discomfort and relieve the pain. Most of all have fun!).

Shiatsu maintains health, vitality and stamina in the body. It strengthens internal organs and prevents energy from getting blocked. Applying pressure to the meridians and chakras opens up the electrical pathways of the nervous system. As you open these points you release negative energy, toxins, or emotions (chemical, electromagnetic energy) which helps us to move with greater ease. The therapist should be sensitive to the patient's emotional, and stress-related work or lifestyle and help to remove the blocks mentally and spiritually that create tension as well.

Acupressure

Acupressure is similar to Shiatsu. In Shiatsu, the practitioner manipulates various parts of the body. Acupressure differs from Shiatsu in that it consists mainly of pressure point therapy. Acupressure requires the recipient's participation with the therapists in coordinating the breath with the manipulations. It is a quiet and contemplative form of massage having profound results. (Like I said, we're all in this together.)

Foot Reflexology

Foot reflexology is a science based on the principle that there are areas in the feet that correspond to every organ, gland and other parts of the body. With specific hand and finger techniques, the feet are "worked" to break down deposits and cause reactions. These reactions could best be described as relaxation, or a return to equilibrium.

Sports Massage

Sports massage focuses on the psychological and physiological effects of exercise. It is geared toward the professional athlete to improve fitness and performance endurance and in the prevention and treatment of injuries.

A holistic practitioner who uses massage therapy may

apply a combination of all of these techniques as needed. There are many books on massage. Check your bookstore and also health food stores for books on massage and healing therapies that are best suited for you. I love you — and me. Here's to many days ahead of happiness, health, prosperity, enjoyment and inner joy.

Love, Peace, Blessings and Smiles.

Hatha Yoga

Hatha Yoga postures (asanas) unifies mind, body and spirit, creating inner harmony and peace. Hatha Yoga emphasizes relaxation as much as it does tension. It conserves energy rather than expends it, for Yoga eliminates excitement which adds toxins to the system.

A few minutes of daily practice in total awareness of body and mind, will ultimately produce a calming state of inner control, a positive mental attitude, and a more energetic and loving spirit.

Suggestions for Yoga Practice

In Yoga, one should never strain. Relax, never force yourself. You will be astonished how many poses you can accomplish by progressively deeper relaxation.

Practice postures out of doors or by an open window. The more fresh oxygen received into the body, the greater benefit derived from the posture.

Yoga should be practiced on an empty stomach or at least three hours after eating.

If you cannot bend your body into a particular position, don't concern yourself, for tomorrow is another day. Now is the time to cultivate patience.

Movements should be slow, but deliberate in every case. Sudden, jerky movements should be avoided.

Before you begin, it is better to wash and attend to your body functions.

Start with a minute of silent prayer, open your eyes or let them remain closed and begin asanas.

The postures on the following page are Yoga asanas which you may use in your private sessions at home.

Stretching the body while using the breath helps to release tension and mental stress, and release toxins out of the body.

Om Shanti (Peace)

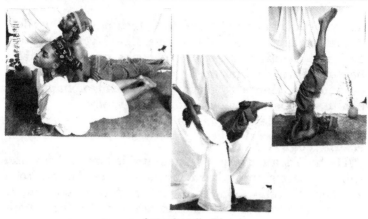

ARI-ANKH KA

Ari-Ankh-Ka is the most ancient form of Afrakhamitic yoga. (Ari = do, make; Ankh = life; Ka+soul). It literally means to make the soul come to life. Illustrations of the postures of Ari-Ankh-Ka have been found on the ancient Khamitic Temple walls. The beauty of Ari-Ankh-Ka, unlike Hatha yoga, is that with each posture there is a specific *Hesi* (ancient sound). This stimulates a greater healing, oneness, inner power and balance (*Maat*) between the various body organs. Ari-ankh-ka was revived in these times by Hru Ankh Ra Semahj Se Ptah, Senur of the Temple of Ptah. Says Senur Semahj, "Ari-Ankh-Ka consciousness affirms our *connectedness* to Divine. While yoga seeks to yoke to Divine, ARI-ANKH-KA IS HU-KA AMI NTR — the authoritative utterance of the soul dwelling in Divine."

An Ancient Khamitic Prayer
Offer yourself up before and after Ari-Ankh-Ka postures.

AMMA SU EN PA NTR
Give praise to the Most High

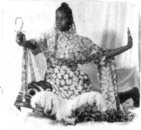

SA-UKSU EMMENT EN PA NTR
Keep yourself daily for the Most High.

AU-TO AU MAAKETI PA HRU
And do it tomorrow as you do it today.

Chapter 17

Holistic Lovemaking

**Diet and Lifestyle in Preparation
for Divine Exchange of Fluids**

Prepare your mate for clean, purified lovemaking 24 hours in advance. Take fruits so she/he will be as sweet as fruit.   If you eat pork or beef, you will have a smell and taste like that of a pig or cow. Instead, eat plenty of watermelon and berries.

Partners: Be considerate. I have already discussed the negative affects of dairy products on women's reproductive organs and the direct relationship between eating dairy products and developing tumors and cysts. Men must also avoid eating dairy, as it produces unhealthy acids and mucus in the semen. A man could end up poisoning the woman he loves while exchanging body fluids during lovemaking.

The same goes for men who interact with women who regularly eat devitalized, mucus producing foods. If her fluids (juices) are impacted with these foods, then her partner's body can become ill, particularly if he is a vegetarian, faster or fruitarian.

The lovemaking experience should be an uplifting one, not a dangerous one. Here is an herbal combination to help you prepare for lovemaking.

For men: Burdock - cleansing and detoxing. Use 3 tablespoons to 3 cups of water.

For women: Red raspberry - rejuvenation of female organs.
Dandelion-healthy blood, physical strength.
Additionally, both can use alfalfa.

Diet 3 to 24 hours before lovemaking should consist of all fruits (with the exception of bananas), salads, and live vegetables and fruit juices. Freshly pressed apple, pear, pineapple, grape, papaya are all sweet nectars that help your body and temperament be as sweet. Remember, foods affect your attitude.

Also take wheatgrass. Stay away from starches, fried foods, meats, and sugar (which destroys nerves, brain, bones and causes stress). Take an enema, herbal laxative or Heal Thyself Colon Deblocker (3 tablespoons with lemon or lime water). Eat lots of okra, a natural laxative. Dr. Moore, may he rest in divine peace, said that okra is good for the male and female sexual organs. It acts as a rejuvenator.

Here is a bath to use in preparation for divine lovemaking. It can also be taken once a week to maintain a sweet, soothing disposition.

Soak individually or jointly with mate in a bath of 2-4 lbs. epsom salt, ½ cup ginger, 2 tbsp. cinnamon and 1 tbsp. nutmeg, a natural bubble bath, and rose petals for 30 mins. Burn non-toxic jasmine in your bath area (hydrotherapy room), if desired. Afterwards, massage one another with sweet oils. Omit the salt if you have high blood pressure.

Heal Your Inner Environment

Don't make love if angry, mad, enraged, or in any adverse emotional state. Your state of mind will be released into your mate who will in turn experience your pain. Meditate or visualize beautiful thoughts and feelings.

Some people take drugs and alcohol to make love, but it destroys the senses, poisons the blood, and invites lower forces (satanic forces) into your union and distances you from the Creator.

As in all things the Creator must be present. So it is in lovemaking. *Note:* If you are free of drugs and alcohol and your partner is not, your pure body will take in your partner's fluids as poison. These toxins will leave the once-pure partner intoxicate, unfulfilled, unhappy and empty of spiritual food.

Heal your lover and heal thyself.

Infertility Among Women and Men

Fast as often as possible (for 7-21 days monthly for 3 to 6 months) to totally restore the reproductive organs.

Clean the colon of old impacted waste that is probably pressing down on your organs and causing blockage.

Lay on slant board daily for 15 to 30 mins. or place face up against the wall in a 45^0 angle with your back facing the floor. This will assist in sending an extra supply of fresh blood and oxygen to the reproductive organs and to allow for a smoother flow throughout your system.

Use Queen Afua's Clay over pelvis of both men and women for at least 3-4 times weekly. Cover clay with gauze overnight. The next morning shower pelvis with hot and cold water (2-3 rounds).

Drink at least 12-16 oz. of carrot, beet, and scallion juice daily. Take the male and female herbal tonics listed in the Nature Cure section.

Restore Lost Fluid in Men after Lovemaking

Women, prepare and serve this formula to him to help prevent premature aging, sexual impotency, prostrate gland blockage, loss of hair and mental deterioration. A constant releasing of sacred fluid without replenishing will cause some or all of the above health imbalances over a period of years.

Formula: 2 tbsp. Lecithin
200 mg. Vitamin E
15-30 mg. Zinc
2 ounces Pumpkin seeds (soak overnight)
8 oz. of Water
Blend together
Raw honey or raw maple syrup, for taste

For additional rejuvenation take saw palmetto berries herb (2 tbsp. with 2 cups of boiling water). Steep 1 hour and drink for extra male potency.

Toward Divine Lovemaking and Conception

Two to three days prior to lovemaking the couple should eat only fresh fruits and raw vegetables, as well as live juices. In the mornings, take the juices of (2) grapefruits and (2) oranges. Take herbal laxative or enemas daily for 2-3 days to unclog the reproductive organs. Take Heal Thyself Formulas I, II, and III, as well as the herbs: Red raspberry, for women; saw palmetto, for men. Add 3 tablespoons freshly pressed ginger with each herb in water.

Fortify with:

- Breathing and exercises: 100 rounds of fire breathing together, two times a day. This will make you more sensitive to one another's touch and thoughts.
- Place legs in 45⁰ angle against the wall while lying on your back for better circulation to the sexual organs.
- Other exercises: squats, leg raises (20-30 times), sit-ups (10-30 times), pelvic lifts (4-10 times).
- While laying on back, inhale and exhale breath with the each movement.
- Cleanse and energize reproductive organs. Do for 2-3 days. Men, apply Queen Afua's Rejuvenating Clay pack over your genitals for one hour, then shower. Women, insert clay 2 inches into the vagina with or without cotton swab; leave for one hour and wash out.

Results:
  ▸ A "sweet" vagina.
  ▸ Your body will smell and taste sweet and clean.
  ▸ More sensitive to one another's needs, thoughts and feelings.
  ▸ You will be more creative, never bored. Boredom indicates you need a great deal of cleansing and

rejuvenating. The cleaner you are, the more creative and loving you are.

▸ No longer will you be exchanging one another's sickness.

▸ Orgasms will be more intense, stronger and last longer.

▸ You will experience the sacredness of lovemaking as a divine and blessed act.

Take a "Love Bath" before union (separate or together):

1 tbsp. Cinnamon
3 tbsp. Rosewater/3 tsps. Rose oil
Natural bubble bath
Handful of patchouli[3]
1-2 lbs. Dead Sea salt (for deep relaxation)
Soak 20-30 mins.
Soft music, small candle, fresh flowers.

Hand scrub body with lemon or grapefruit while in tub. Take shower afterwards. (This step is optional for extra pure skin.)

After bath:

• Dry and anoint your mate with rose water or oil. Use musk (men); sandlewood (women), or other uncut pure oil of your choice.

• Sprinkle cinnamon around the sheets (according to the late Dr. John Moore).

• Boil 1 teaspoon of cinnamon or nutmeg in a pot of water, to bring a sweetness into the air of your home temple.

I recommend that you don't make love in red or black or hot pink, for it evokes only stimulation of the lower chakras. Work with the colors that are listed in handbooks

---

[3] Jackson, Judith. *Sensual Touch*. N.Y.: Ballentine Books 1986. p.25

to help stimulate the 4th (heart) to 7th chakras (crown, spiritual).

Don't make love haphazardly. Prepare yourself and your environment for such a divine interaction. While making love, have thoughts of giving, exchanging beauty, respectful, spiritual, healing and nurturing. Know that you both are a gift from the Creator to one another. High thoughts, purified feelings and cleansed body temples bring forth a healthy, loving and spiritually advanced child to the world through you. The baby is a reflection of the couple. Preparation for conception should be three months to one year living on a system such as described in this book.

Love taboos: Never make love when confused, angry, tired, guilty, depressed or weak, for you will poison one another through your imbalanced devitalized fluids and weak spirit state. When in this state, make love by long walks in the park, embraces, hand-holding and candlelit dinners to strengthen relationship and self first.

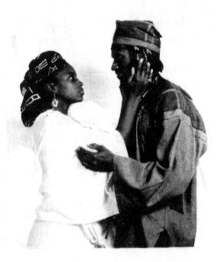

Spiritual Union

Mundane loving is not all there is. While making love, be tender, be powerful, be sweet and oh so gentle. Chant together. As you move, breathe in and out in sheer harmony. Whisper words of peace, joy and contentment.

During love-making, and particularly during your divine orgasm, visualize what goodness you desire for your mate and go so far as visualizing the beauty and healing your desire for the planet on which you live; for the burning fire within us is now activated and potent to move out into the Universe by way of your third eye and crown and heart chakra.

Women, say while in your lover's arms: I am a divine temple and I will you most divine love. When you enter into my temple walls I will transform you and renew you. When you enter my gate you will find peace, for I am pure love. You may enter, my gentle strong king man.

Man, say while in lover's embrace: I am a divine DJED (Afrikan-Khamitic word meaning stability) designed for your sacred garden. As I enter my djed into your great temple walls, I come with a scepter of transformation, balance and high direction. My coming to you will bear you gifts of deep beauty and warmth, protection and peace. Allow me in, my precious queen woman so that we may travel the galaxy as one.

And when you join together and travel through many pylons and doorways to arrive at the shore of that vast ocean of bliss, as you ride on that Great River together, an inner explosion occurs and the heavenly gates open within you, ushering a oneness upon you. Remember that moment of stillness, of splendor and tranquility, and absorb that oneness into your life as transformative healing, for your union when pure in heart and body is a gift supreme from God to you. **Note: This level of love-making is almost impossible if you consume the flesh of an animal or devitalized food and drink. Men, if you persist in a destructive diet, prove your love for your mate by wearing a condom.**

On Finding Your Soul Mate

To attract a divine mate you must become divine in your state. I bear witness to countless testimonials from students and devotees of cleansing who found their soul mates. Others have healed their broken marriages by living and loving in the ways of purification.

Remember, it can happen in the twinkle of an eye or during a 21-day fast ... so fast and pray and fast and pray.

Then one day in your divine state, a reflection of a mate will appear before your very eyes if only you would purify.

So light a pink candle and go your way and know that he/she will be coming any day.

May This Love Last Forever

The love that we exchange, let it last forever. Let love inspire, encourage, strengthen and nurture us. Let this love last forever. Let that love be within the baby that we created so beautifully; that idea that we created so brilliantly. Let love last forever, and with each love experience let it be a lesson, a blessing, a teaching, a sharing. May this love last forever.

In Celebration of Our Men

A Love Letter

I love you, Black Man, Afrikan Man, Khamitic Man.
    We, Afrikan Women, love our men.
Our union's endured through the storms, pains, pressures
    & hardships that kidnapped us to these shores.
Hundreds of years have gone by yet we still maintain our
    deep love for you, even when we have been separated.
In the quiet night, I called out for you.
    Did you hear me?
I know you can feel me.

I love you... I've loved you from the beginning
    And I will love you for all eternity.
Nothing, not even time will stop me from loving you
My love for you is unshakable, unbreakable, unconditional
    and simply — age-less.

You are the first man, the finest man, the most regal.
    All men after you use you as the example of Manhood.

My king, scholar, leader, physician, architect, builder,
   lover
You are the Father, the Big Baba of the Earth.

Your Afrikan Women rise up to embrace,
   to cherish and to nurture you.
My beloved King, you have been wounded; you're bleeding
   Sound out the horns! Alert the women and children!
The planet is in trouble.
   The planet will not be right until you, I, we, heal.

"Are you all right?" she whispers.
I will patch your wounds with herbs — comfrey, red clover.

   I will bathe you in hyssop.
I will anoint you with frankincense and myrrh.
   I will feed you with sweet nectar.
I will help us both to heal.
   So many hundreds of years have gone by.
Now take me, rock me in your ancient arms
   and let me know all's right
Make my burden light.
   Let me rest in your mighty bosom and
become empowered by your touch.
   Let me know that all is ALL RIGHT

I need you, for your presence makes me feel like
   the burst of the sun's energy.
What joy, what peace, what pleasure, what comfort you
give to me when you're loving me.
Oh, how my Moon loves to dance around your Sun!

   Black Man, Afrikan, Khamitic Man...
You are to me the bright star that glitters in the night.
   Oh, how I love to touch you, and one thousand stars fill
my soul with pure ecstasy.
   Your strong, loving arms open the heavens for me.
In return I open my heart to you.
   Take care of my heart.

I sometimes sit and think to myself with a smile
  on my face
I can see you in my mind's eye — the Third Eye
  You're as sweet as brown cinnamon, as strong and as
powerful as an oak tree, as firm as a rock ...
  Yet as gentle as a dove.

I thank the Creator with every breath of my being
  for having such a Divine and Noble Reflection.
Oh how we love our King Man.
  Can't nobody love you like we love you.
I love you now, I loved you then, and I will love you
  for all eternity
For our love is unshakable, unbreakable, unconditional
  and simply ageless.
Age-less, age-less... .

• • •

Write your mate a love letter for love heals all wounds.
The greatest Medicine is love, the greatest honor is love.
Love will be showered upon you if you give love. If love is
pure and real it will last forever. If you are not receiving
love, then you have not been giving it. Write yourself a
love letter and bring yourself fresh flowers. Speak words
of love; feel and think thoughts of love. Become love and
you will draw love unto yourself. The greatest, most
perfect love is the love we receive from the Creator. Love
is a gift, a blessing. If you have it, share it. If you want it,
give it.

The Holistic Family

Traditionally, when a member of the family or tribe was
ill, the whole family healed as a unit. It was never just an
individual effort. Every thing was done collectively.
Individualism and separation from family has caused
illness and need. Here are some family healing suggestions
to help regain the natural ancient Afrikan Principles.

Suggestions for Healing the Family

All families should select one day a week for "Family Healing Day." On that day the family does the following to prevent sickness and family disharmony. Take an herbal laxative the evening before "Family Healing Day" so that everyone purges by morning.

- Take an enema with the juice of a lemon or lime added (2 quarts for adults and 1 for children) and a 2-4 lbs. salt bath. The cleaner each family member becomes, the better the communication, the sweeter the dispositions, and the more patient you will be with one another.
- Eat only live fruits and vegetables and drink 8-16 oz. each of the fresh fruit and vegetable juices.
- Participate in family morning and evening prayer, as well as shared affirmation and thanksgiving.
- Wear white or family color of choice that supports your purpose
- Instead of watching TV, make a family video or write a family play.
- Massage one another from head to toe. Use olive oil. If you have aches and pains use peanut oil.
- Do a family clay and air bath, for 30 minutes — this should be healing fun.
- Have a Family Herbal Tea Party. Chat and Enjoy each other. Bring fresh flowers to the home. Clean the house as a family unit.
- Say loving words to one another all day. Carry this family activity over the week in time, but always keep at least one day a week for family unity, bonding, and exchange of beauty and harmony. For without a family there is no civilization. Include your extended family in the love process as well.

Chapter 18

We Are The Elements

The body is made up of all the elements that are present on the Earth. As a result, we must use those natural elements that are in nature to Heal Ourselves: air (lungs), fire (blood, reproductive organs), water (90% of the body consists of this element alone), earth (bones, teeth) and ether (spirit).

As we use the proper elements that are on earth for the healing of our body elements then we will be in total harmony with ourselves, nature, the universe and all our relations. Refer to the following chart as you seek to balance a particular element within the body.

The planet Earth is polluted and all its people are constipated with old, impacted, undigested food and bad thoughts. Everyone have one or more of the elements in their body temple blocked with sickness and disease. Enemas, colonics, drinking large amounts of water, fasting and herbal purges will heal all the sick, tired and over--abused body elements. Once your body is totally cleansed then you are living the ancient quote, "Cleanliness is next to Godliness." Until your body becomes totally pure and free of all disease created by man, then you will never truly be one with the Creator of the Universe. Suffering will continue to be rampant throughout the land. Follow the Element Chart to re-establish your seat in the high council of Natural Living.

FIVE ELEMENT CHART

Using the Angels: Earth, Air, Fire, Water, Ether (Spirit) for Natural Healing.

Employ this chart to help you maintain your health balance.

	Anatomy	Foods	Colors	Physical Activities	Creative expression
ETHER	Head (Mental & spiritual center)	Honey, Fruit	White/black Purple	Meditation Visualization Instrument	Zither/harp Flute/string
AIR	Respiratory/ Nervous system	Sprouts, Leeks, Scallions, Garlic Radishes	White/blue	Hatha Yoga Tai Chi, Ari-Ankh-Ka	Singing Flute Air exercise
FIRE	Reproductive organs Blood stream	Beets, garlic Red grapes, ginger Radishes, cayenne	Red/Orange Yellow	Jogging Aerobics	Violin Drums
WATER	Urinary tract Bladder	Cucumber, Parsley Watercress, Spirulina Blue green manna Grapefruits	Blue/Green	Swimming Sailing Water-skiing	Piano/Flute Painting String instruments
EARTH	Bile/bones	Carrots, potatoes Brown rice	Brown, Black, Green	Biking, Walking Jogging	Afrikan dance Martial arts Drums, Sculpting Gardening

	Emotional Blockage	*Emotional Harmony*	*Physical Diseases*
ETHER	Feeling disconnected from the Creator; Unable to hear your inner voice	Happiness, balance, in tune with the Creator; able to hear your inner voice	Depression, Headaches Lack of creativity
AIR	Quick to judge; stifled and trapped; lacking in patience	Creativity, ability to move freely with ideas and concepts as well as physically and emotionally	Asthma; colds
FIRE	Lack of inspiration, Anger, rage	Joy; being inspirited to live more fully	High blood pressure, fevers impure blood, poor circulatio
WATER	Suppressed need to cry; Feeling overwhelmed Sadness	Harmonious, at peace	Water retention, Edema, Kidney failure, Frequent urination
EARTH	Not being able to progress Inability to move forward; not sharing; feeling overwhelmed	Progressive, giving	Constipation, Tumors, Cysts

	Nature Cures	*Candle Locations*	*Colors*	*Herbs*
ETHER	Visualization Color Therapy Fasting, Crystal Healing	Botanical gardens Mountains	White/purple	Gota-Kola, Vervain Blessed Thistle
AIR	Pranayama (breathing exercises), Air Baths, Sauna, Sun Baths	Parks, Wide open spaces	White	Apple cider Vinegar Eucalyptus Camphor oil
FIRE	Hot tub bath Steem bath	New York City (fast paced, but be aware of burnout), Hot climate	Red (energizer) Blue (calms energy or burn out)	Gota cola Golden seal
WATER	Colonics Baths, Enemas Nose rinses, Fasting	Oceans, Pools, Jamaica or any tropical island	Blue	Chickweed Fennel Bladderwrack
EARTH	Clay packs (internal and external) Bentonite, Crystal, Healing	Beaches parks, Afrika	Green	Cascara, Sagrada Senna, Peppermint

Chapter 19

MESU HRU
The Canopic Jars

The TWA/ANU people of the Nile Valley were the ancestors of those who later formed the great united nation of Tawi. They preserved in their resting places a guide by which we of the present time can maintain our health. Maintenance of health precedes healing as an ideal, for in maintenance we *sustain* the balance. In healing, we seek to *restore* the balance.

We know the adage that prevention is better than cure. Those items that were preserved in the resting places in the Valley of the Kings and Queens are very important for us in these times to know about and to study. For while we may argue that some kings and queens of the nation of Tawi died at a fairly young age, the fact should be remembered that not all of us who have the information on health practice the information. As it is today, so it was then. But the information is still available and if applied, can have a profound effect on the maintenance of health within the body-temple.

The jars that were found are now called canopic jars. These were four jars which contained the lungs, the liver, the small intestines and (combined into one jar) the stomach and large intestines. Our early ancestors (another way of saying "we" in our more ancient phases), placed on the top of each jar the head of an animal, one jar had the head of a man.

In the resting place of the Boy King, ATEN-RA-TUT-ANKH, who is now called King Tut, we find what we believe here at the Shrine/Temple of Ptah to be a revelation that we of the present time can be guided by. This revelation is of great importance because that young

King's resting place was the only one found intact in modern times. The majority of what was found is still preserved. Revelation tells us that the preservation of this vital resting place of King Tut is for us his brothers and sisters in these times — a time capsule that we can consider and use for the reclamation of our Khamitic heritage and legacy. A reclamation of this legacy must begin first of all with the recognition that we have become a sick people and the first business is to heal ourselves.

We cannot seek to change the condition by which we've become surrounded unless we begin with self. We are off-track because of the ingestion of the wrong diet imposed upon us by foreigners. And so that's the reason why this information was all the more important for the initiate. It served to preserve him in a state of health in order to combat the conditions that were pressing in on us then, as they are now. The jar that contained the lungs in King Tut's resting place was positioned on the eastern wall of the tomb. So to us this is a revelation that the east is a place of beginning as we go in a clockwise position. On the eastern wall is represented the guardian Hapi and the face used to cover this jar was the cynocephalus baboon (see Fig. 1). This was one of the so-called sacred baboons and associated with the Ntr *Tehuti*, who is the guardian of letters, of intelligence, and the keeper of time.

In the beginning we said that these heads were chosen because each head indicated that principle for which the organ was created and by which it can be maintained. The baboon urinates every hour on the hour, so its head was used to be an archetype of periodicity. This brings to mind that our breaths are likewise numbered. We must in cadence practice breathing, which is called in yoga — pranayama. Hapi's color is black to indigo. The colors of the blossoms of the herbs can be used to target the specific organ and maintain it in health. Furthermore, we may choose licorice, comfrey root and others to maintain this organ. Those herbs that will support the element of air are the herbs that we should ingest for the maintenance of this guardian. A guardian is a servant, like an angel, and as such in the Afrikan context must be fed its proper food.

As we now come to the south we have *Qbsenuf,* the guardian of the small intestine (Fig. 2). Qbsenuf's animal is the falcon. We know that the blood consumes its food through the walls of the small intestine and thus the nourishment is transferred along this passsage. The nourishing chyle is offered to the blood as sustenance and this then aids the warrior within to conduct the battle of another day. Of course, we know that the falcon is commonly referred to as a warrior bird, and it has always been the perennial symbol of the Khamitic royalty of Tawi. The keen vision of the bird is also very well known. Among hunters, it is used in the art of what they call falconry. Hence our ancestors chose this bird to indicate the spirit that comes from the food fed to this organ; the spirit of speed, of deep piercing sight, ascension to spiritual heights, which the falcon exemplifies.

The color for the guardian of the small intestine is white, and as such, the foods are garlic, ginger, etc. It is at this point that the water is literally wrung out through 26 feet of intestines. This guardian's element is water and it would require us to consume water to help to maintain the fluidity and peristaltic activity of this organ.

As we move to the west, we find the guardian here has the face of a man and he has the name Amset (Fig. 3). This is the guardian of the liver. His color is green, which refers to the bile and also to its opposite (yellow) when the liver is vexed. The yellow indicates jaundice.

This is one of the most important organs in the mainte-nance of the cleanliness of the blood and so it must be fed its proper food and maintained in a state of calm. The liver is known to register the emotions of the individual and so the face of a man was put on it because in the face we can read the condition of one's liver. A calm face would indicate that the liver is likewise, calm, and is being properly maintained. It is on the face that the emotions are mainly registered. This guardian rules the element, earth.

The jar with the head of a jackal represents *Tuamutf* and the cardinal point, north. He presides over the functions of the stomach and large intestines. The food in the stomach is in a partial state of digestion. We should say that it begins at the very thought of eating because the salivary glands begin to do their work in preparation for the breakdown of food in the mouth. The stomach, the pouch at the bottom, catches what we ingest.

This is the place where the food goes through the most pronounced function of digestion because it's here that the digestive juices (enzymes, acids and alkalies) come in to aid this process to make it easier for the small intestines to assimilate and also a place where further digestion takes place. It's possible that toxins can escape through the walls of the large intestines and cause further vexation to the blood. *So it is important that peristaltic action of this organ be kept in tone with fire foods that we find the color red ruling.* The foods that have blossoms and seeds of red are particularly good for maintaining the health of this organ. Cayenne pepper, sorrel, watermelon, beets (preferably when young to lessen the amount of starch), and other foods that have red in them will aid in the maintenance of the fires of Tuamutf.

Hapi — is the name of the river which we call the Nile today. It is associated with the bull because the river in its inundation was seen as a bull — strong, vital and regenerative. Hapi is also the name of the constellation which we now know as Aquarius. Hapi is the Khamitic name and sound. In this age the element of air rules and Hapi is the ruler of the lungs. We are bombarded in this age by the impurities in the air, and so it is important that we feed detoxifying foods to Hapi to reduce the damage of modern life.

Qbsenuf — the name means "he refreshes his brethren." The refreshment is the nourishment of the foods going to the blood stream. The name envelopes this principle in action.

Amset — the very name means green. This is the seed of nourishment. It is also the place where the youth of the body can be maintained. We target purifying foods for the liver. Bitter foods correspond with the substance produced by the liver.

Tuamutf—means "to praise." "Mut" means mother, "F" is the personal pronoun "his." He praises his mother, the fire from the energy that comes from the divine. Mother is the topsoil which delivers the vegetation that we take in for the nourishment of the body. The stomach literally praises this divine principle.

Sound is also very important and vital to the maintenance of these organs. These names, when uttered, tone the respective organs.

MESU HRU
(The Canopic Jars)

FIGURE 1   FIGURE 2   FIGURE 3   FIGURE 4

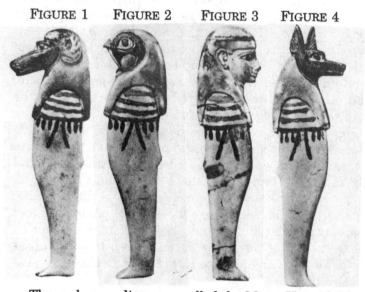

The male guardians are called the MESU HRU (children of Hru). The female nurturers are MUTU EM MESU HRU (mothers of the children of Hru). These female nurturers that stand guard over the male neteru are Nebt Het over Hapi, Serkhet over Qbsenuf, Ast over Amset, and Net over Tuamutf. Feed them with herbs and evoke their names for "toning" of the organ with sound vibrations. HRU (You) are the immaculate Divine Child born of the union of AST (mother principle) and ASR (father principle).

HRU ANKH RA SEMAHJ SE PTAH

THE KHAMITIC ELEMENT CHART FOR HARMONY

Neteru	Figure 1	Figure 2	Figure 3	Figure 4
Direction	East	South	West	North
Male *Guardian* Female	Hapi Nebt het	Qbsenuf Serkhet	Amset Ast	Tua-mut-f Nt
Organs Guardian Task	Lungs Breath-regulation	Sm. intestine Absorption	Liver Blood-purification	Lg. intest. /stomach Digestion/ egestion
Color	Black/indigo	White	Green/yellow	Red
Herbs	Licorice, comfrey ...	Garlic, ginger, etc.	Mints, etc.	Cayenne etc.
Element	Air	Water	Earth	Fire

Chapter 20

Spirituality

**A Cleansed Body Temple Is
A Prayerful One, So Fast And Pray**

To cultivate tranquility, harmony, love and health, let life be a prayer. Your every word, movement, thought, your comings and goings, your joy, your sadness, your inhalation and exhalation, your every breath, your work and play, let it all be prayer. For in that continuous prayer you shall be lifted into heaven on earth. Your body temple will become one of pure light and love, which is God. When you live in this natural divine way, a golden stream of blessings continually flows your way. There, no disease can be found; only health, wealth and happiness abound. So fast and pray. Fast and pray. Pray all misery away.

As you *prepare* your juices, let it be a prayer. As you *drink* your juices and herbs, allow them to flow through as you fill up with light and love. With each drink, see your aura change from brown, black and gray to blue, pink, green, and white. See yourself become illuminated, moving beyond the Earth's plane. See that sacred nectar transform you to where you know you should, could, and must be.

As you rise at dawn and rest at sunset, let it be a prayer. As you cleanse your home, your temple, your sanctuary, let it be an act of worship. As you sit, stand, walk, let your prayers come through.

As you "be" love, as you make love, offer it all up in prayer. Then and only then will all that you do and say be protected from all harm, all hurt, all darkness. There is no darkness in prayer, only the light of the Creator. So fast and pray; pray your misery away.

Devotion to Purification
as a Spiritual Path

When you are cleansed or are a "Devotee/Initiate of Purification," you no longer resort to destructive behavior such as through the use of self-abusive elements, i.e. alcohol, drugs, tobacco, gossiping or complaining. Instead, you follow the "26 Laws for Devotees of Purification as a Spiritual Path." Practice the following — exercise, take walks, salt baths, or showers. Drink glasses of warm water or a Heal Thyself Nutritional Formula with juice. Pray or meditate. Fast on fruit and vegetable juices. Give thanks and praise. Each time you choose this progressive response/action, you climb higher and higher into your spiritual and physical self-healing. It cannot be said enough. A Devotee of Purification is one who will purify at all costs. Regardless of what is going on in their lives, they will cleanse. If upset, take a bath. If you have lost your mate, cleanse your home. If lacking money, wear green, light a green candle and pray. If confused, take gota-kola and do shoulder or headstands.

26 Laws For Devotees Of Purification

1. Fast and purity for all seasons, conditions and circumstances.
2. Pray daily as the 3 cycles of the sun are being ushered in.
3. Maintain clean thoughts, heart, and feelings at all costs.
4. Fast and purify on your personal Holy Day and your community's Holy Day.
5. Live by the *Heal Thyself* text.
6. Woman: fast during your menses or eat only live foods. Men: during your mate's menses, fast and pray with her for divine harmony and a cleansing of the relationship.
7. Free yourself from disease of the body temple, heart, and mind.
8. Become a vegetarian, fruitarian, or liquidarian.

9. Do not use drugs, alcohol or engage in out-of-season lovemaking.

10. Follow the Dietary Timetable that is ruled by the sun.

11. Begin a fast or purification ritual with every seasonal change, with every new moon (for 24-36 hours) to affirm new dreams and prayers.

12. Silently meditate every full moon period. Take green juices and rejuvenating herbs during this time for inner peace and balance (Maat).

13. Pray daily for universal peace and purification for yourself, for family, nation and world.

14. The clothing you wear must reflect the beauty and harmony seen in nature and the oneness with the Holy Spirit. Use color charts to assist your choice as to what you want to express to the world and attract or repel from you.

15. Support all those in their healing who request your assistance in some way, big or small. In this way you support yourself.

16. Use the four elements to heal yourself daily.

17. Become active in spiritual and community work of your choice.

18. Give self-less service/aid to someone less fortunate than yourself as often as possible, or at least during every new moon period.

19. Once a month fast for 24 hours abstaining from all foods, liquids, sleep and lovemaking.

20. Show love, give love, and appreciate love with and from your birth family, extended family and all your relations.

21. Be the first to ask for forgiveness; be the first to forgive.

22. As a city dweller, go to rest in parks, or by the ocean to recharge your spiritual and physical self.

23. As a country dweller, be blessed to be able to visit nature daily.

24. Let your home be your temple, your sanctuary. Purify it daily with water, frankincense and myrrh, sage and cider.

25. Recognize cleansing as a spiritual practice our
    ancient ancestors used as a rite of passage for initi-
    ates into higher understanding and the Mysteries.
26. Listen inwardly for total guidance every step of the
    way.

Daily Spiritual Purification Discipline

1. 6:00 Sun Rise
    Recite Water Prayer (see *Hydrotherapy*) while tak-
    ing shower or bath. Dry your body and put on white
    attire before going into prayer.

2. Sit on chair or pillow (*Be sure to open a window in
    the room in which you are praying.*) Perform the
    Breath of Life Exercises:
      25-100 Cooling Breaths
      100 Fire Breaths (500 Fire Breaths for work).
    Sing or chant/spiritual songs or chant the universal
    sound "OM." "ANKH."

3. Read a passage from your personal spiritual book.
    For example:
    Hu Sia
    Holy Bible
    Book of Coming Forth into Day from Night
      (misnomered The Egyptian Book of the Dead)
    The Upanishads
    Essene Gospel of Peace
    Holy Qu'ran
    Kahlil Gibran's *The Prophet*, etc.

4. Activities of Prayer Session
    (a) Thanksgiving
    (b) Prayers
    (c) Forgiving
    (d) Affirmations

5. Song/Chant i.e., "fasting and cleansing"
    After chanting, go into meditation for 5/30/60 mins.

6. Become the Ocean of Life
    Set up a simple altar comprising:
    - one glass of water to absorb negative vibrations
    - a spiritual book
    - crystals to purify and charge the area
    - pyramid (optional)
    - fresh flowers
    - picture of spiritual teacher in this world or the
      spirit world (your ancestors)
    - cloth to cover low prayer table
    - candle 15 hours or 7 days (Place candle in a glass
      bowl.)
    - Burn non-toxic incense of jasmine or frankincense
      and myrrh with charcoal to purify the home.

A FASTING POEM

Confessions of a Low Vibration Junkie

Day breaks!
Got the Shakes!
Mind slipping...
Nose dripping
Body aches

I feel real bad, like the flu,
I got the detoxification blues ...
Got an attitude.
Feeling bad.

Want some fried chicken, Mad...
you see, you see
"My Jones is coming down on me."

Why won't these toxins let me be.
I want to be free, free, free.

Ringgggg, ring, ring — "Yes, Queen Afua I know; take

two enemas and call you in the morning."

Bacon, eggs, cheese on toast.
Mmmmmmmmmmmm, yea, yea ... No!
It's really pus on toast
Mucus on toast.

The Last Poets
That doesn't sound good
I'll eat/drink what I should

Yea, some Lecithin, Spirulina, TwinLab,
And of course the carrot-beet.
Mmmmmm, yea that should put me on my feet.

Now I'm ready to hit the street ...

But the situation remains ...
and it's plain ...
and it be ...

My Jones, my Jones is coming down on me.

Got to change my mind set
Got to get on the positive bet

Negative thought I must defeat
My constitution must be complete
I will eat to live
Not live to Eat!!!
The path towards purification
Lays at my feet
and
me being me
Black, down, and determined to be free
Will not, will not give into my vulnerability.

There is no road too arduous for me.

My vulnerability is only a state of mind.

My "Jones" a part and parcel of the disease.
True change/revolution can only be effective at 360^0

"Free your mind"
Your ass will follow
Heal My Self as I should

I will endeavor, the very best I can, and
To quote the Most High — God
"It is good!"

Roger Moore,
A 21-day Faster.

Heal Thyself Formulae
For Fasting and Healing

Your general nutritional supplement is Spirulina or
Wheatgrass (powdered), or a more potent 1-2 oz. of liquid
Wheatgrass. Take 1 tablespoon of Spirulina, wheatgrass
or Queen Afua's Super Nutritional Formula I three times
daily with juice. If you have a chronic disease, for intense
rejuvenating take 1 tablespoon of both Spirulina and
Wheatgrass. If you feel nausea after taking this combination, reduce the amount by one-half. Once your body is
cleansed you will be able to handle the chlorophyll, and
you will be able to take larger amounts of green drinks (as
much as up to 2-3 tablespoons of either or 2 oz. of fresh
pressed wheatgrass).

Take Vitamin C in the form of lemon, lime, grapefruit,
rosehips tea, cayenne pepper, or Vitamin C 500-1000 mg.,
twice a day, up to three times a day when fasting. Heal
Thyself health products are geared towards achieving
health through *nutritional* fasting and *natural* healing.

Queen Afua's Super
Nutritional Formula I

The Super Nutritional Formula of Wheatgrass and
Spirulina is an almost complete food. The addition of
psyllium aids in the elimination of old impacted waste
trapped in the colon.

Formula I contains:
   Vitamins A, B_1, B_2 -Folic Acid, B_3 -Chlorine, B_5 -Inositol,
   B_6, B_{12}, B_{17} (the entire Vitamin B complex), Vitamins C

(ascorbic acid), E, F, K, Potassium, Copper, Iron, Calcium, Chromium, Magnesium, Manganese, Sodium, Molybalenum, Zinc, Phosphorus, Selenium, Silicon, Cobalt, Sulfur, and trace minerals.

To prepare Formula I:

☞ Blend and drink promptly 1-2 tbsps. Formula I with fresh fruit or vegetable juice 2-3 times daily.

Take B Vitamins for anti-stress. If you have skin problems or a nervous condition take 2 tablespoons of chlorophyll in addition to B vitamins. If problem persists after a week or two, add TwinLab Yeast without the whey (liquid form from 15-50 mg.) For best results, contact a nutritionist, a naturopath, an herbalist or holistic health consultant to give you the personal guidance you may need. Use the above information as a general guide.

Queen Afua's Master Herbal Formula II

The Master Formula II contains 13 powerful herbs designed to strengthen and cleanse every system within the body temple. (Number 13=4. The number 4 represents building, in this case, building a strong body temple).

Ingredients include:

1. Gota-Kola - brain food.
2. Comfrey healing and knitting of bones. This herb food is excellent for male and female productive organs as well as a bladder and kidney tonic. Comfrey is high in calcium.
3. Alfalfa - builds and strengthens. It contains Vitamin A, E, K, B and P. Alfalfa contains protein, phosphorus, iron, potassium, chlorine, silicon, magnesium and sodium and has within it 8 enzymes which promote chemical reactions that enable food to assimilate within the body.
4. Echinacea - blood cleanser, antiseptic, reduces glandular swelling.

5. Blessed thistle strengthens the heart, liver, lungs and kidneys.
6. Red Clover - blood purifier, anti-cancerous herb, soothes the nerves and rejuvenates the gall bladder.
7. Cascara Sagrada - relieves chronic constipation; intestinal tonic; assists in cleansing the liver.
8. Mullein - valuable in asthma and lung affliction. Aids in calming the nerves. Aids in eliminating ulcers and tumors.
9. Chickweed - excellent for weight loss. Aids inflamed eyes and skin disease. (The late Dr. John Moore recommended this herb to help burn excess fat.)
10. Dandelion - purifies and helps to neutralize the acids in the blood. It eliminates anemia, aids in skin disease, such as jaundice and eczema. It is useful in relieving kidney conditions.
11. Ginger - to increase circulation and to expel mucus congestion.
12. Chaparrell - an anti-cancer herb.
13. Fenugreek - clears mucus from the bronchial passages and has a healing effect on the bowels.

To prepare Formula II:

☞ Boil 4-5 cups of purified or distilled water. Turn off boiling water and add 4-5 teaspoons of herbal mixture (Formula II). Allow it to steep over night. Strain in the morning. (Use the leftover herbs in a bath and soak.) Do not reheat or refrigerate. Drink from morning to 12 p.m. (High Noon) for freshness and potency. Take 5-7 times a week.
Note: Vitamin D, T and U, although not in Super Nutritional Formula I, are contained in the Master Herbal Formula II. Vitamin P (Bioflavonoids) can be acquired from the white inner skin of lemons, oranges, and grapefruits. Iodine can be obtained from kelp, watercress and artichokes, to name a few sources.

Formula III — Colon Deblocker

The Colon Deblocker contains 3 potent cleansing oil to lubricate and detoxify old impacted waste from the colon. *Ingredients:* Castor oil, cold pressed olive oil and Vitamin E.

To prepare Formula III:

☞ Take 2-3 tablespoons of Formula III daily with the juice of 1 lime or lemon, or with kidney-liver flush, first thing in the morning. Take every other day when fasting. Take 1-2 times a week while on the Natural Living Program.

A Word To The Healers

Healing was a very sacred work in ancient times. The healing arts were reserved for priests and priestesses, medicine men and women, "bush" doctors and other people who were respected for their knowledge in the sacred mystery systems.

Likewise, healing is also a very sacred work in this present time when this planet and its people are in serious need of healing — spiritually, mentally, physically, educationally, economically — in short, totally.

When the three main aspects of the human body are aligned and in proper order, we feel at peace. We are then in a state of well-being. We are able to function on a much higher octave mentally, physically and spiritually.

However, when these three major aspects of the body are out of order or alignment, there is then a malfunctioning and the individual needs healing, realignment and rejuvenation. When any of these areas are out of order they affect the other areas. Body areas are interrelated and have some definite effect upon each other.

Often times when people go to the hospitals for treatment the doctors focus on their physical ailments and never look into the mental or spiritual discord which perhaps could be the root of the illness in the first place. When there is some mental disorder detected, patients are sent to psychiatrists, psychologist and others who focus on mental disorders. Patients are sent to different specialists who handle only an aspect of the person's problem(s). As a result, people may be left feeling disoriented or dissected.

Healing, on the other hand, is meant to bring the person into a state of oneness, order and balance; to bring all of the different aspects together in harmony. True healing comes from the Creator and thus when we are living the natural laws and in tune to the Creator and the natural laws of the universe we are healed. We are at peace within our lives.

Medical doctors have taken oaths to live up to their profession and to execute the best service they can with the knowledge that they have acquired. It is also the responsibility of the healers to live up to a high moral code and to be good examples of a what a healed person is before they can begin healing treatments on others.

We realize that the oath of healers must include being clear clean vessels so that the Creator can work through us to help to heal others. How can we expect to heal others if we ourselves are out of order mentally, physically, and/or spiritually.

Our first responsibility is to heal ourselves so that we may become shining examples of positivity, of intelligence, of love, of cleanliness, of strength, of kindness, of right thinking and right action, for these are aspects of the Most High that are associated with true healing.

I remember times in the past when I hesitated going for spiritual readings or healing because the practitioners themselves did not look healthy or happy, positive or pure. This made me feel that whatever reading I got could not be a higher vibration than the person delivering the information. In relation to this, no matter how wonderful a beautician may style your hair the vibration of the beautician is still upon your head.

This message to healers emphasizes that no matter how long you have been practicing your particular craft, all that is not of the Most High will be exposed eventually, for "no lie can last forever."

Perfect healing consists of 360° of healing — body, mind, and spirit. Until the healers incorporate this complete formula for healing their clients and in their own lives, they will always find something is still missing. The healing will still be incomplete.

Let us surrender ourselves to the Master Healer and ask to be forgiven for our shortcomings. Let us humble ourselves so that we may be truly uplifted in the pure light. We will thereby walk with a glow and radiance around us. We will be holy in spirit so that we may be true servants of the Most High. We wish to be used to help heal our people and this planet in truth, and in righteousness, in the name of the Most High.

Queen Esther
Co-Director of Heal Thyself Center 1987-1989

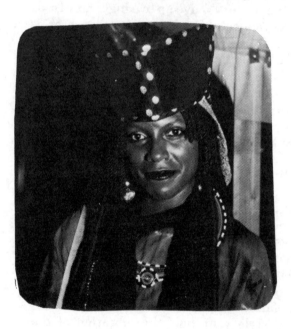

Chapter 21

Testimonial Declarations

Fasting, through the Heal Thyself Center, has positively changed my life. I've been spiritually, mentally and physically healed and empowered. Tapping into a higher consciousness is now more easily accomplished. My key words are now — *fast and pray.*

Sandra Watson
Director Family Institute for
Edition, Training and Employment
La Guardia Community College, CUNY

In the Khamite legacy, Asar (Osiris), Lord of Regeneration, manifests as Hapi (the river Nile) in its inundation. Periodic inundation, through colonic water cleansing, along with herbal ingestion is the greatest tonic for body and mind. I can attest to the fact that water purification and cleansing as I have experienced at Heal Thyself with Queen Afua has been beneficial and in tune with my Khamitic orientation.

Hru Ankh-Ra Semahj Se Ptah
Sen-ur of the Hetep Ptah Temple

When I went to Queen Afua, my legs were so bad that I could not walk without thick pantyhose on. I took the 21-day fast in June and now my legs feel so good. I just rub my legs and thank God and Queen Afua for their help.

Rachel Franklin

When I was a child in Afrika I dreaded the inner cleansings my mother would treat me to. It is a form of enema called *asa* in my language, Akan of Ghana. This treatment prevented my brothers, sisters, and myself from being sick. At the first sign of constipation, headache, stomachache and other ailments *asa* was prepared and administered. Unpleasant as it was, that was what kept us bright-eyed, strong and healthy.

Inner cleansings have been an ancient health practice of Afrikans since time immemorial. It was after I started having colon irrigation recently, as an adult, that I confirmed this ancient health practice of our ancestors. My eyes are brighter, my sight clearer, I am much healthier all the time, my joints are stronger and I never even catch a cold in this treacherous ecology. My creative level and energy level is so high that I feel reborn.

To the Afrikan, health is inner cleansing and eating healthy. It is law: the law of nature. It is for the birds and the entire animal kingdom. The birds by divine intuition know what seeds and leaves or herbs to pick and digest.

Divine intuition is supreme law. Intestinal cleansing is the guaranteed way to a vibrant healthy life.

Joe Mensah

Fasting has touched all aspects of my life — mental, physical spiritual. Physically, it gave me the opportunity to cleanse my body in preparation for the child I was to conceive. It was not a planned conception, but a truly divine conception. One year to the day I undertook the first of four 21-day fasts, not realizing the Creator was preparing my body for the birth of another spirit returning.

Mentally, fasting has allowed me mental clarity; it removed a lot of mental pollution that clogs us all. It gave me the opportunity to be still and make decisions and choices that had eluded me for years. I finally was able to make the step to economic freedom and the creation of my own law firm with my brother.

Spiritually, it led me further down the path of our divine state. It brought peace, balance, patience, and forgiveness into my heart.

Yet fasting is as unique an experience as each of us is unique. The particular benefits of a fast may be seen immediately or manifest slowly. A fast is the creators tool to bring us to divinity.

Universally, fasting purifies a nation, a world. Remember Gandhi freed his people with fasting! Peace.

Dianne Ciccone
Esq. (lawyer)

When I first heard about Heal Thyself, I was 35 years old and about 20 pounds overweight. I also had fibroids on my uterus and lumps in my breast which became painful every month before my menstrual cycle began. In addition, I was beginning to develop lines on my forehead and was chronically fatigued. Like most women my age, I accepted these conditions as my lot, ... part of being thirty-five. Then I saw my neighbor, a female around my age, and she looked fantastic! Her skin was clear and glowing, and she looked about 10 years younger than the last time had seen her. ... I was in Queen Afua's office less than a week later and I joined the 21-day fast the following week. Within 21 days I lost 21 pounds and the lines in the face were gone. I went to the doctor and was told I had no fibroids and the lumps in my breast were gone. Needless to say, I continued to follow a vegetarian diet and now fasting is a part of my life. People cannot believe that I'm 40 years old; they guess my age to be around 25. I have got more energy than I had when I was 20. A typical day for me starts at 5 a.m. with jogging. I go to work, do all of my housework, laundry and cooking for my family, and go to the gym most evenings. I've also joined two community organizations, something I never was able to find the time or energy for. I no longer bleed every month and the doctor says that my blood count is higher than the average woman's. Every day I thank God for Heal Thyself and I've encouraged all of my friends and family to take advantage of the many benefits this program has to offer.

Judy Shepherd-King

Praise the Lord for Queen Afua and her wonderful staff at Heal Thyself. Richard and I started the 21-day fast on

Sept. 11, 1989 and successfully graduated Oct. 1, 1989. I had the urgency to continue the fast, so without a break I continued the next 21-day fast, further experiencing a renewal and cleansing that I find extremely difficult to verbalize. During all this time I was receiving regular colonics, steam baths, body massages, following instructions from Heal Thyself, having full emotional and physical support from my husband and drinking large quantities of NSA water.

As the second 21 days began to come to a close, I still had the need to continue — without a break — to a the third 21-day fast. During the entire time, I worked everyday and had only a 1-day crisis. The only area that I had not followed was the instructions of taking the Sonne 7 and 9. For the last seven days, I have taken the Sonne and the results have been awesome. I now understand that cleansing never stops — and we won't stop!

Verran Barter

Before I went to Queen Afua I was always tired/sleepy. I had no energy. When I decided to go on her 21-day fast, I followed the instructions carefully. Now I feel great, wonderful. I've never felt better in my life. I have a lot of energy. I feel stronger. My skin looks younger, softer and smoother. I can think clearly, and I understand better. I communicate better with my husband and children. I am more relaxed. I can deal with any type of problem, even those I could not deal with before.

I would like everyone to know that I lost 22 pounds in the course of the fast. I am ready to go on the next 21-day fast. I am even planning on becoming a vegetarian. I have not eaten meat in 6 weeks. Again, I feel wonderful and great. I want to thank the Creator for guiding me and keeping me strong so that I could go on with this fast. I want to thank Queen Afua for helping me get through my fast. While fasting I prayed to the Most High for healing. I now want to make this my lifestyle forever.

Bayanah Robinson

Name: Withheld by request.
Occupation: Withheld by request
Illness: *Drug Addiction*
Length of time: 10 years

During the 21-day fasting program I was able to overcome the desire for drugs. From the first day on the fast I felt a spiritual healing and physical cleansing unknown to my being. I knew I was truly healed when I could walk pass the drug spot and have no desire for some, whereas prior to the program the need, the desire, and the addiction was ever-present. Thank you. Peace & love.

Name: Nazlah Hudgins
Occupation: Baker
Illness: *Trance Seizures*
Length of time: 5 months 5/89-10/89
Drugs taken during illness: None

In March 1989, Nazlah began laughing in an uncontrolled manner which gradually led to trances seizures. At the time she had a seizure she was able to hear me, however, she would stare around, play with her fingers, and/or pace back and forth.

After consulting with Queen Afua, she began a nutritional program of solely live food consisting of leafy green salads, freshly squeezed oranges, carrots and beets. In addition, Nazlah was fed fresh fruit, herbs and vitamin supplements.

Approximately 2 months after consulting Queen Afua, the trances ceased.

Name: Sameerah Sabree
Occupation: Manager
Illness: *Tumor on right breast*
Length of time: 1954-1985
Dugs taken during illness: Herbs

In 1954, I entered high school. I then discovered a

blackhead pimple on my right breast. After I squeezed it, it became to grow into a lump that was eventually larger than a chicken's egg. Doctors wanted me to have the lump removed, but I kept putting it off because cancer runs in my fathers and mothers families . I refused to be "knifed." I did have a cancer test, but I tested negative. I went on worrying through life about my condition, hoping and praying that this lump would go away someday.

Well, about April 1985 I was introduced to the Heal Thyself Center in Brooklyn, NY. This was the beginning of a new life for me. I was introduced to the method of herbal treatment. I first started with the colon cleansing, vitamins, herb teas, exercise and fasting. After 2½ months of this method I was then given the pack for the breast. The remedy for the breast was to use once daily castor oil, green clay and hot heating pad, so this could loosen up the lump. Not until the last 2 weeks in July did something happen. One night this lump burst while I was asleep. When I woke up that next morning I was faced with a new life. This was the greatest experience I have ever felt. It was as if I had released a 40-pound bowling ball from my stomach. I'll always be grateful to the managers and to God for this time of my life. Three months of healing. Thanks.

Name: Deborah Jordan
Occupation: Word Processor
Illness: *Overweight / headaches*
Period: Overweight — past 2 years; headaches as long as I could remember.

I am very thankful for Heal Thyself because for as long as I could remember I have been getting (suffering from) terrible headaches. Since going to them the headaches have eased up considerably and I have lost weight on the fasting program and am continuing to do so. I will continue going to them to receive advice on good eating habits and on my health.

Name: Angela Terrick
Occupation: Nurse's Aide and Student
Illness: *High Blood Pressure, Asthma, Abdominal pain*
Length of time: 8 years

I am grateful and thankful to the Heal Thyself group for healing my sick body with their prayers and herbal treatments. For 8 years I suffered with an asthmatic condition, high blood pressure and abdominal pains. As a result of the treatment program I have made great physical improvement. I no longer suffer from asthma, high blood pressure or abdominal pains. Now I am enjoying excellent health.

Name: Joan F. Alexander
Occupation: Telephone Operator
Illness: *Menstrual problems*
Period: 5 years

I was sick, disgusted and frustrated with pain month after month, taking pain killers (600 mg. Motrin). I was introduced to Heal Thyself Natural Living Center. During my visit to the Center in Sept. 1985, I underwent a healing process in my body that doctors could not do for me. The pressures and pains I previously suffered had been very intense. But thanks to a wonderful friend of mine who kept pushing me to go to the Center, I am satisfied with my healing and I am enjoying my life once more. Thanks be to God the Father, and his Son, Jesus Christ, who can always make the impossible possible. With God, all things are possible. I do hope that more people will start understanding that where doctors fail Heal Thyself will prevail.

Name: Ethlyn Olyna Jordan
Occupation: Clerk
Illness: *High blood pressure and Arthritis*
Period: 20 years

In one week or less after starting this fast, all of my arthritis pains were gone. My blood pressure was down to

130/186 from 180/110. Thank God for Heal Thyself Natural Living Center.

Name: Thelma Halstead
Occupation: Classroom Teacher
Illness: *Anemia / anemia-related symptoms*
Length of time: Over a period of years

Thelma Halstead affirms that she attended the Heal Thyself Center from July 1985 to the present time, March 24, 1986. She has received colon therapy (cleansing), nutritional advice and fasting therapy (consultation). During this period, she received remarkable alleviation of these health problems — anemia, enervation, lassitude, cystitis, intestinal gas, and narcolepsy.

Name: MaryLee Miller
Occupation: Teacher
Illness: *Hormonal imbalance and fatigue*
Length of time: 7 years

My healing experience began in 1986. During the first 3-4 weeks I spent 21 days fasting and cleansing internally, as well as externally. Many of the symptoms of my hormonal imbalance have disappeared: fatigue, dry skin, menstrual problems, headache, lower back pain. I have stopped taking the synthroid and no effects have come up. The herbs I'm taking are correcting the problems that in the past have come up in this situation.

Epilogue

Purification Oath

Go tell it on the mountains; go tell it everywhere, that purification is here for I am purified.
   I am purified
   I am purified.

Forgive me, I will be a sinner no more.
I will not defile the gift the Creator
has bestowed upon me.
I will cleanse and build a body temple of light, for am purified.
   I am purified
   I am purified.

Give me the power and strength to release that which brings about Satanic reaction and action. Release me from eating pork, beef, all flesh, milk, cheese, ice cream, fried foods, and sugar. Free me from my tumors, my cysts, my high blood pressure, aches and pains. Release me from the strong grip of alcohol and drugs. Free my soul from these desires. For the fall of humankind was ushered in hand-in--hand with these dark tools, and the purpose was destruction.

I cry out, RESURRECTION. I AM the resurrected. Creator, help us to turn our backs on darkness and direct us to the Truth and the Light. Help us to use the divine tools of inner freedom. Show us the joys of eating foods made by your hands. I say "Yes" to fresh fruits, vegetables, sprouts, whole grains and herbs. For it is said, "behold, I have given you every herb-bearing seed which is upon the face of the earth, and every tree, in which is the fruit of a tree yielding seed; to you it shall be for meat.

167

Let it be known that through the hands of purified souls, bodies and hearts a New Age will ushered in. Personal, collective and global resurrection begins when we have the power and the faith to accept your divine, unchanging path of purification.

Burdens of envy, pain, hate, anger, rage, lust, jealousy, lack and limitation, today, are no more in my life for I am Purified
    I am purified
    I am purified.

Love, joy, abundance, peace, gentleness, health and wealth are mine for I am purified
    I am purified
    I am purified.

My blessings, my gifts, my hopes, my dreams, my freedom awaits me. Let the heavens and earth rejoice. I am one of the Chosen Ones, for I am purified.
    I am purified
    I am purified

Let purification ride on wings of air.
Let purification ride on the ocean of Life.
Let purification shine from the blazing sun.
From me to you and you to me.

Yes, go tell it on the mountains.
Go tell it everywhere, that the Creator is here to let everyone know that fasting, prayer and purification is the way, and you must come through the door of purification to reach God-realization today.

Yes, go tell it on the mountains. Go tell it everywhere Rejoice that purification is here
    I am purified.

    I am purified.
    I am purified.

Creator, Neter, Jah, Jehovah, Allah, God Almighty, Krishna, Yahweh, Yeshua, Olodumare, I'm home. I've come home to my original purified God-like state. I am purified.

I am purified

I am purified.

Queen Afua

TO ALL MY RELATIONS, TO THE PEOPLE MENTIONED
HEREIN, TO ALL MY CLIENTS, MY FRIENDS, LOVED ONES
WHO HAVE COME INTO MY LIFE, AND I INTO THEIRS.

A Love Poem

We have exchanged healing through the years
I pray our love has grown potent enough to travel on the
winds of our dreams and our realities
I pray our love will be felt in the spirit even when we are
unable to hear or see one another

What peace, what joy we would feel all the time
For this deep love knows no bounds, no limits
I love you my blood and extended families for all the
lessons, challenges, and blessings received through you
I love you for being the Creator's co-pilot and for helping
to make, shape and mold me into a healer
Or better still, a vessel of healing
For the Creator is the Grand Master Healer.

We are the vessels that the Holy Spirit (Neter) chooses to
work through if we are but willing to serve.
I love you for helping to make me grow even when you
weren't conscious of your assistance in my evolution.

There is no sadness in my years;
Only tears ... of joy and understanding
Only bliss — memories of the peace, strength, courage and
soul-searching knowledge we shared.

"No man or woman is an island."
It takes all of us to make you, and all of you to make me.

* * *

In Celebration of Our Children

This written word was inspired on July 24, 1991, at 5:43 a.m. as I was giving thanks and praises for my children whose entire life from birth to now has been a sacrifice, because of my 24-hour commitment and dedication to my life work, Healing. These words are also in honor to all our children everywhere.

Don't grow up with overt or suppressed anger about your parents. Know that we love you, know that we love you in different ways; so that when you grow from a seed to a tree you will be without resentment, which is illness. You will be a whole, healthy and beautiful tree. Forgive us for all inconsistencies and mistakes and lack of knowledge about parenting. Forgive us for being preoccupied with the world's problems and overwork and constant worry about your future. I know we will strive to be there for you at times when you need us most. We vow now as parents of the planet to do better, to be more balanced in our decisions about life, and you. Keep in mind just as you as are a child growing daily, moment by moment, so are we as parents growing moment by moment into wisdom and understanding. Let us extend patience to one another, parent to child. Let us continue to grow into greatness of unconditional love: for my love of you is deeper than my soul, and stronger than my own flesh.

We, the Parental Community of the World, vow to guide, love and protect you. We vow to bestow a blessing upon you such that as you go daily into the world no danger will befall you. We vow to aid your growth with life-giving and life-sustaining, natural foods. We vow to keep your body free from fast foods, i.e., fried burgers, soda and other artificial foods that slowly kill and destroy your body, spirit and mind. We will keep you free of flesh foods that makes us sometimes behave in a deadly way and age us before our time.

We vow to fill you with fresh herbs, vegetables, whole grains, live juices, sun-ripened foods made by the Creators hands. Each portion of food you take into your body temple will not only feed your body but feed also your spirit.

We, as Parents of the World, vow not to poison you with violent TV. viewing or micro-dinners, or physical abuse in word or deed or glance.

As your mother (mama) I vow upon your coming to this earth to feed you with breast milk and comfort and love so that you will receive the divine nectar that was ordained for you.

As your father (baba), I vow to be there for you in sickness or health; during life and beyond death.

We vow as parents to be your Nature care practitioners and to use (4) elements to heal you and keep you well from so-called necessary childhood dis-eases of mumps, measles, chicken pox, earaches, hyperactivity, colds fevers and runny noses, and from bad dreams.

We vow to support and nurture the special gifts you come to share with this planet.

We vow to praise all your good deeds for none are too big or too small. We vow to set good example so that you can grow strong, confident and stable.

We vow to teach you the spiritual ways so as to repel darkness and draw a life of light, peace and joy unto you.

There is an Afrikan proverb that says, "*It takes a whole village to raise a child.*" My prayer is that through our continued healing of thyself our love enlarges such that we can receive a continuous and abundant love from one another.

I love you for helping me to write the pages of my life in its many shapes and colors through the eyes of a healer.

Lovingly,

Queen Afua

Queen Afua

WEEKLY HEALTH CHECK LIST

FOR NATURAL LIVING NUTRITIONAL PLAN
(Indicate dates in columns provided)

Photocopy this chart or use as a guide for creating one of your own.

1	Shower - alternate hot and cold. Or 4-8 lbs. Epsom salt or 1-2 lbs. Dead Sea salt in bath.							
2	Prayer / Meditation							
3	Pre-Breakfast (Kidney-liver flush)							
4	Exercise (15-30 mins.) Begin with 50 full body breaths and 100 rapid fire breaths.							
5	Breakfast (juice if fasting)							
6	Lunch (juice if fasting)							
7	Dinner (juice if fasting)							
8	Tonic (finish by 12 noon) before tonic spoils)							
9	Read books on Natural Healing or Spirituality 30 mins. daily							
10	House Cleansing (House fast)							
11	Nutrition (taken 2-3x a day with juice or water)							
12	Live juice (take 2-3x a day)							
13	Nose Rinse (use netipot or teapot, add a pinch of sea salt to water and cleanse nostrils)							
14	Enemas or Herbal Laxative							
15	Queen Afua's Cleansing/ Rejuvenating Clay							
16	Hot oil packs with Castor oil (use for tumors, cysts especially)							
17	Total self-massage (Reflexology)							
18	Prayer/Meditation/Visualization Exercises							
19	Be loving to self and others							
20	Talk Fast (indicate hours) for spiritual strengthening and focus							

Chart 1

Heal Thyself Purification Wheel

The Small World vs. The Larger World

Cleanliness is next to Godliness/NTR. Purification is holiness, as in wholeness, as in healed. Because the Creator represents all that is whole, as you dedicate, commit, devote and discipline yourself daily to purify from within, all areas of your divine being will be made holy (whole), stable, full of brilliant light, surmounted with the love of the Creator. Purification is the way of the Most High. You represent the light of the Most High. For each light that is lit moves us closer to planetary salvation. As you graciously accept Natural Living & Nutritional Fasting as a way of life, all the many parts of you will be made whole.

As illustrated with the Purification Wheel, you will see that the Microcosm births the Macrocosm into reality. To alter the macrocosm you must alter the microcosm, by purifying from within. As we reach up the ladder of **P** (Purification) and **R** (Rejuvenation), P + R = *Maat* (Balance), which = Health in Body, Mind, and Spirit. We mold our world daily, for true change begins from within. To the extent you use the Resurrection tools is the extent to which your larger world broadens, heals, and transcends to the highest degree.

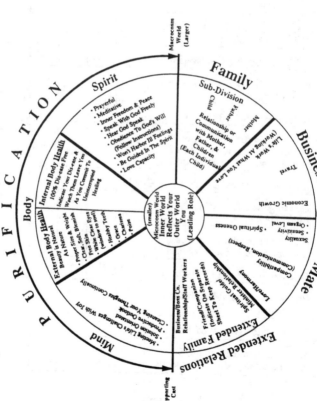

Chart Your Course To Success with this "Total Life Healing Chart"

Chart 11

PURIFICATION CHART (Sample Diagram)

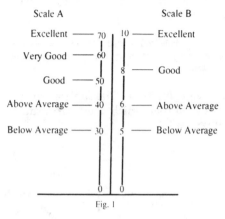

Read your score from fig 1 and place it in the chart fig. 2.

Δ Let the spirit guide you, chart yourself by way of initiation (your inner feelings)

Δ Score yourself monthy to chart your progress

Δ Repeat this (12) week cycle for one year for P.H.D. of Purification.

Δ Every 3 Months reevaluate your progress & continue the process of growth; while charting your way to a life healing.

Δ If you keep close to the Heal Thyself method of Natural Living and Nutritional Fasting you should experience within the 1st month a 60% improvement, by the 2nd month 80% , by the 3rd month 90-100% improvement. After the 3rd month its all about maintance of the natural living laws in order to keep a consistant high life rating.

Fig. 1

The (12) Week Cycle to Restore & Purify Your World

Use scale B to access ones states of being and fill in the number in fig. 2. Use scale A to rate ones total. The total is the sum of ones state of being ratings for an entire month. Score from the point you begin. Evaluate every 30 days whether your point of start is in the beginning, middle or end of the month.

Example:	Mind	Body	Spirit	Family	Extended Family	Business	Mate	Total	Remarks
Beginning of the First Month	5	4	7	2	2	6	5	31	Below Average
End of the First Month	8	8	7	6	6	8	10	53	Good
Second Month	8	9	7	7	7	7	7	52	Good
Third Month	9	10	9-10	9	9	10	10	66.5	Excellent

Fig. 2

A word to the wise on the Purification Charts for support in working with these unique charts it is advised to take the (four) week Heal Thyself Natural Living and Nutritional Fasting course so that you may Learn how to effectively chart yourself to success.

Layout by Mast Djed Nefer Publishing

Chart 111

YOUR TOTAL LIFE PURIFICATION CHART

FILL IN THIS CHART AS A HEALING MEDITATION ACCORDING TO YOUR NEEDS

As you work on your chart your meditation is as follows: As I Purify from within I Heal and Purify from without, and all the parts of me that make me whole and free!"

"To the Yogi the entire universe is his body. The Matter which composes his body is the same as that which constitutes the universe."[1]

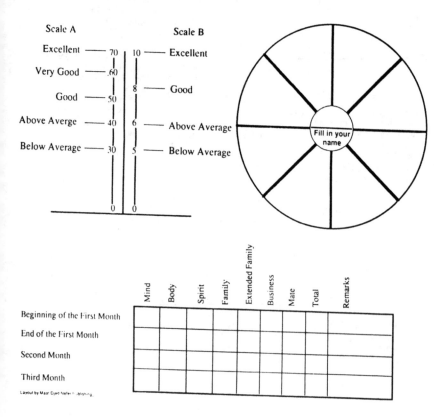

[1] Swami Sivananda *Science of Yoga* vol. 12 pp. 5-6.

RESURRECTION TOOLS AND METHODS

As you use any of the Purification Tools, energize the action with words of power and healing:

"FASTING AND CLEANSING"
"FASTING AND CLEANSING"
"FASTING AND CLEANSING"
"LIBERATION THRU PURIFICATION"
Chant 4 times for all four corners of the universe

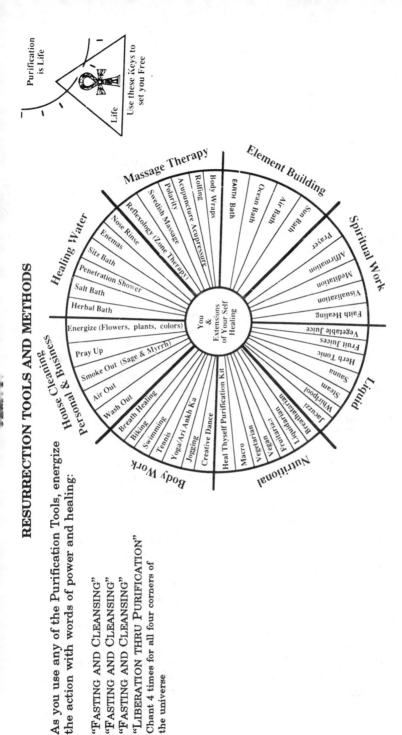

Purification is Life

Life

Use these Keys to set you Free

House Cleaning
Personal & Business

Natural Living and Nutritional Fasting are the foundation of the various other methods that you use to support your resurrection. For cultural healing contact Sen-ur Heru Ankh Ra Semahj of the Shrine of Ptah   *Charts I-IV courtesy Maat Djed Publishing*

177

Index

Selected Bibliography

Cunningham, Scott. *Magical Herbalism*. New York: Llewellyn
  Publications, 1989.

Dextreit, Raymond. *Our Earth. Our Cure*. New York:
  Benedict Lust Publication, May 1974.

Dufty, William. *Sugar Blues*. New York: Warner Books, 1975.

Ehret, Arnold. *Mucusless Diet Healing System*. Beaumont,
  CA: Ehret Literature Publishing, 1972.

Gregory, Dick. *Dick Gregory's Natural Diet for Folks Who
  Eat: Cookin' with Mother Nature*. New York: Perennial
  Library, 1974.

Jackson, Judith. *Sensual Touch*. New York: Ballentine Books,
  1986.

Kirschmann, John D. *Nutrition Almanac*. New York:
  McGraw-Hill Book, 1975.

Kloss, Jethro. *Back to Eden*. New York: Beneficial Books,
  1972.

Kulvinskas, Viktoras. *Survival into the 21st Century*.
  Woodstock Valley, CT: 21st Century Publications, 1975.

Muramoto, Naloru. *Healing Ourselves*. New York: Avon
  Books, 1973.

Parvati, Jeannine. *Hygieia: A Woman's Herbal Book*
  Berkeley: Freestone Collective, 1978.

Rose, Jeanne. *The Herbal Body Book* New York: Grosset &
  Dunlap, 1976.

Szekely, Edmond *The Essene Gospel of Peace Bk.1* Matsqui,
  B.C., Canada: International Biogenic Society, 1981.

Walker, Dr. Norman W., *Colon Health* Prescott, AR: Norwalk
  Press, 1970.

Walker, N., D.Sc. *Diet and Salad*. Prescott, AR: Norwalk
  Press, 1974.

Walker, N., D.Sc. *Fresh Vegetable and Fruit Juices: What's
  Missing In Your Body?* Prescott, AR: Norwalk Press, 1970.

HEAL THYSELF PROGRAMS

- Private Holistic Health Consultation
- Dietary Instruction or Supervised Fasting.
- Health Evaluation.
- Pendulum Reading of the Body Systems.
- A Nutritional & Herbal Program will be developed for your maximum potential weight loss. Gain improved health with knowledge received within this session. Spiritual Guidance, as needed.
- Personal Tape of Session included (if requested).
  Total: $55.00

21-Day Fasting Program

Workshops on the principles.

Group and/or private consultation with Queen Afua, before and after workshops.

21-Day Heal Thyself Supply Kit with includes: Nutritional Herbal Formulas, Colon Deblocker, Personalized Guidance and Heal Thyself Manual and Journal. Queen Afua is available for seminars at your church, business or organization, as well as for radio or TV appearances on the following topics:

- Fasting Seminars.
- Natural Living Seminar for the Entire Family.
- Sacred Women's Training.
- Bless Your Disease Away.

Her office hours are Monday, Wednesday and Friday from 10-6 p.m. Call for an appointment at (718) 953-0009

Heal Thyself with Queen Afua's
Product Line for Natural Living and Fasting

Kits

Home Study Project Transformation Program: A 3-Month
Holistic Weight Loss and Natural Living Lifestyle Program
Includes Formulas, Tapes and Booklets . . . . available

Heal Thyself Holistic Health Kit
Includes: Formula I - Super Nutritional, booklet, journal
            Formula 2 - Master Herbal, tapes, herbal pack
            Formula 3 - Colon Deblocker & Cleanser
21-Day Supply Kit. $ 195.00

Healing Products:

Heal Thyself Rejuvenating Clay   (8 oz.) . . . . . $ 15.00
                                 (4 oz.) . . . . . $ 10.00

Literature & Cassette Tapes

Heal Thyself for Natural Healing and Longevity $ 9.95
Master Your Health with the How, What and
Why of Fasting   (90 min.) . . $ 10.00
Natural Living for Purification and How to set up your
   Home as a Healing Center   (90 min.) . . $ 10.00

Buttons and Bumper Stickers

"Liberation through Purification" . . . . $ 1.00

Heal Thyself Holistic Health Home Video Course $ 95.00
                              (Four VCR Tapes)

Please mail money order to:

HEAL THYSELF CENTER
323 STERLING PLACE
BROOKLYN, NEW YORK 11217

Or, for pick-up of orders, call Queen Afua at:
(718) 399-1903